ANIMAL MODELS AND HYPOXIA

RELATED TITLES OF INTEREST

Books

I. HANIN & E. USDIN: Animal Models in Psychiatry and Neurology
J. SKODA & P. LANGEN: Antimetabolites in Biochemistry, Biology and
Medicine

Journal

Biochemical Pharmacology

ANIMAL MODELS AND HYPOXIA

Proceedings of an International Symposium on
Animal Models and Hypoxia, held at Wiesbaden,
Federal Republic of Germany, 19 November 1979

Editor

V. STEFANOVICH
Hoechst, Wiesbaden
Federal Republic of Germany

PERGAMON PRESS

OXFORD · NEW YORK · TORONTO · SYDNEY · PARIS · FRANKFURT

U.K.	Pergamon Press Ltd., Headington Hill Hall, Oxford OX3 0BW, England
U.S.A.	Pergamon Press Inc., Maxwell House, Fairview Park, Elmsford, New York 10523, U.S.A.
CANADA	Pergamon of Canada, Suite 104, 150 Consumers Road, Willowdale, Ontario M2J 1P9, Canada
AUSTRALIA	Pergamon Press (Aust.) Pty. Ltd., P.O. Box 544, Potts Point, N.S.W. 2011, Australia
FRANCE	Pergamon Press SARL, 24 rue des Ecoles, 75240 Paris, Cedex 05, France
FEDERAL REPUBLIC OF GERMANY	Pergamon Press GmbH, 6242 Kronberg-Taunus, Hammerweg 6, Federal Republic of Germany

First edition 1981

British Library Cataloguing in Publication Data

Animal models and hypoxia.
1. Brain chemistry - Congresses
2. Energy metabolism - Congresses
I. Stefanovich, V.
591.1'88   QP 364.7   80-41991
ISBN 0-08-025911-1

In order to make this volume available as economically and as rapidly as possible the authors' typescripts have been reproduced in their original forms. This method has its typographical limitations but it is hoped that they in no way distract the reader.

Printed in Great Britain by A. Wheaton & Co. Ltd., Exeter

PREFACE

In the second half of the twentieth century study of brain metabolism has grown into an important scientific discipline with many talented and diligent investigators from various fields working toward a common goal. This extraordinary development has resulted in a series of information contributing to the understanding of various aspects of brain metabolism and function.

And still it appears that a systematical evaluation of a series of experimental animal models employed to study brain metabolism in various physiological and pathological situations is rather insufficient.

To increase our knowledge and to offer a review of the different animal models concerning brain energy metabolism in general, and hypoxia in particular, the Symposium "Animal Models and Hypoxia" was held at the Nassauer Hof, Wiesbaden, on November 19, 1979. This Symposium was also the result of the understanding that large meetings are non-optimal means of a communication within specific areas of a biomedical research. Small symposia, where extensive discussion is limited to a selected number of participants with leading authorities in the particular scientific area in attendance, are recognized today as an optimal means for the exchange of information. The Symposium "Animal Models and Hypoxia" was also designed to encourage participant interaction by alternating presentations by invited speakers with round table discussions. All in attendance were invited to freely and informally exchange thoughts and ideas.

The publishing of the Proceedings of this Symposium is the result of the conviction that the lectures presented on this occasion, deserve a much wider audience than was represented at the Symposium. Each chapter in the book reviews a particular subject in detail - from the regional utilization of glucose in the brain of mammals, by Dr. Sokoloff, to energy metabolism in the nervous system of insects, by Dr. Wegener - giving a valuable information on the available knowledge to date. It is expected,therefore, that this book will have a wide reading audience.

It is also hoped, by the editor of these proceedings that the animal models, suggested in various chapters, can also be useful in the search for a new medicine. The discovery and development of a new drug is a very difficult, complicated, expensive and time-consuming process. Hopefully, this book will be of some help in this area also.

At the end, the editor would like to express his gratitude to the contributors for their excellent work, time and help, to all participants for a stimulating discussion, to the publisher, especially Mr. M. J. Richardson for his cooperation, and to Mrs. H. Felke for her secretarial assistance.

V. STEFANOVICH

v

CONTENTS

Opening remarks   viii
  E.WOLF

Mapping Local Cerebral Functional Activity by
  Measurement of Local Cerebral Glucose Utilization
  with the [^{14}C] Deoxyglucose Method   1
  L.SOKOLOFF

Energy Metabolism in Isolated Rat Brain   19
  J.KRIEGLSTEIN, B.DIRKS and J.HANKE

Animal Models in Experimental Gerontopsychiatry   35
  S.HOYER, L.FRÖLICH and M.HOF

Experimental Occlusion of the Middle Cerebral
  Artery in Cats   47
  K.-A.HOSSMANN

General Discussion   59

The Role of Sympathetic Innervation in the Regulation
  of Cerebral Blood Flow During Hypercapnia   65
  O.HUDLICKA and C.T.HING

Chronic Normobaric Hypoxia and Subcellular Isoenzyme
  Patterns of Rat Brain Lactate Dehydrogenase   75
  H.H.BERLET, V.STEFANOVICH, B.VOLK, T.LEHNERT
  and M.FRANZ

Comparative Aspects of Energy Metabolism in Nonmammalian
  Brains under Normoxic and Hypoxic Conditions   87
  G.WEGENER

Anoxic Rat Model   111
  V.STEFANOVICH

Index   125

OPENING REMARKS

I am greatly honored and very pleased to welcome you on the occasion of the symposium "Animal Models and Hypoxia". I got very enthusiastic when I learned that a workshop conference on the mentioned topic should take place. I think we face a strange situation: There is an increasing number of elderly people. Recent surveys showed that the number of people over 65 years of age in the United States is increasing at an annual rate of nearly 400.000, making this the most rapidly expanding segment of the population. The situation in Europe is similar.

In addition, it is estimated that the elderly use 2.2times more drugs than their younger counterparts. On the other hand, the drug developers are accused of ignoring the elderly. Whether or not this really true, remains open for discussion, although there is no doubt that we live in a century which does not favour the elderly. "Old is not beautiful". But it goes without saying that we lack active drugs for the treatment of the aged. This, however, has nothing to do with the lack of interest, but it reflects the fact that it is extremely difficult to establish reliable animal models. I do hope that this symposium is a step forward to develop appropriate animal assays which correlate with the human disease.

E. WOLF

Mapping Local Cerebral Functional Activity by Measurement of Local Cerebral Glucose Utilization with the [14C] Deoxyglucose Method

L. Sokoloff

Laboratory of Cerebral Metabolism, US Department of Health, Education and Welfare, Public Health Service, Bethesda, Maryland 20205, USA

ABSTRACT

A method has been developed to measure the rates of glucose utilization in the individual structural and functional components of the central nervous system. It can be applied to conscious as well as anesthetized animals. The method is based on the use of [^{14}C]deoxyglucose as a tracer for glucose consumption. [^{14}C]Deoxyglucose-6-phosphate accumulates in the tissue in a mathematically definable relationship to the rate of the tissue's glucose utilization. The [^{14}C]deoxyglucose-6-phosphate concentrations in the various tissues of the nervous system are measured by a quantitative autoradiographic technique. The autoradiographs themselves are pictorial representations of the relative rates of glucose consumption in these tissues. Application of this method to rats and monkeys in various physiological, pharmacological and pathological states demonstrates a clear and close relationship between the local levels of functional activity and energy metabolism. The method appears to be useful for mapping functional neural pathways on the basis of evoked metabolic responses and for identifying loci of actions of pharmacological agents.

KEYWORDS

Brain metabolism, glucose utilization, deoxyglucose.

INTRODUCTION

The brain is a complex organ composed of many structural and functional components with markedly different and independently regulated levels of functional and metabolic activity. In more homogeneous organs that do readily recognizable physical and chemical work, such as the heart, skeletal muscle, and kidney, a close relationship between functional activity and energy metabolism is well established. The existence of a similar relationship in the tissues of the central nervous system has been more difficult to prove, partly because of uncertainty about the nature of the work associated with nervous functional activity, but mainly because of the difficulty in assessing the levels of functional and metabolic activities in the same functional component of the brain at the same time. Pathological and pharmacological conditions with gross and diffuse effects on cerebral functional activity, particularly those that alter the level of consciousness, have been shown to be associated with changes in overall cerebral metabolic rate (Kety, 1950, 1957; Lassen, 1959; Sokoloff, 1976), but such associations could reflect separate independent consequences of cellular dysfunction rather than a direct relationship between cerebral functional activity and energy metabolism. Changes in the metabolic rate of the brain as a whole have generally not been found during physiological alterations of cerebral functional activity (Lassen, 1959; Sokoloff, 1969, 1976). What has clearly been needed is a method that measures the rates of energy metabolism in specific discrete regions of the brain in normal and altered states of functional activity. The recently developed [^{14}C]deoxyglucose technique (Sokoloff and colleagues, 1977) appears to fulfill this need. It can be used to measure quantitatively the local rates of glucose utilization simultaneously in all the macroscopically visible structures of the brain. It can be applied to normal conscious animals as well as those under experimentally altered states of cerebral activity. Furthermore, the [^{14}C]deoxyglucose method employs an auto-radiographic technique which provides pictorial representations of the relative rates of glucose utilization throughout the various components of the brain; even without quantification these autoradiographs provide clearly visible markers that map cerebral regions with increased or decreased rates of energy metabolism in altered physiological, pharmacological, and pathological states. This method has provided unequivocal evidence of a close relationship between functional activity and energy metabolism in discrete structural and/or functional units of the nervous system.

METHODOLOGY

A full, detailed, and comprehensive description of the theoretical basis of the [^{14}C]deoxyglucose method has recently been published (Sokoloff and colleagues, 1977). A brief summary of its essential principles is necessary, however, to clarify the salient features of its design, its rigid procedural requirements, and the limitations on its applications.

The method was designed to take advantage of the extraordinary spatial resolution afforded by a quantitative autoradiographic technique that was originally developed for the measurement of local cerebral blood flow (Landau and colleagues, 1955; Reivich and colleagues, 1969). The dependence on autoradiography prescribed the use of radioactive substrates for energy metabolism, the labeled products of which could be assayed in the tissues by the autoradiographic technique. Although oxygen consumption is the most direct measure of energy metabolism, the volatility of oxygen and the short physical half-life of its radioactive isotopes precluded measurement of oxidative metabolism by the autoradiographic technique. In most circumstances glucose is almost the sole substrate for cerebral oxidative metabolism, and its utilization is stoichiometrically related to oxygen consumption (Kety, 1957; Sokoloff, 1976). Radioactive glucose is, however, not fully satisfactory because its labeled products have too short a biological half-life and are lost too rapidly from the cerebral tissues. The labeled analogue of glucose, 2-deoxy-D-[^{14}C]glucose, was, therefore, selected because it has some special biochemical properties that make it particularly appropriate to trace glucose metabolism and to measure the local rates of cerebral glucose utilization by the autoradiographic technique.

Theory

The method is derived from a model based on the biochemical properties of 2-deoxyglucose (Sokoloff and colleagues, 1977). 2-Deoxyglucose (DG) is transported bi-directionally between blood and brain by the same carrier that transports glucose across the blood-brain barrier. In the cerebral tissues it is phosphorylated by hexokinase to 2-deoxyglucose-6-phosphate (DG-6-P). Deoxyglucose and glucose are, therefore, competitive substrates for both blood-brain transport and hexokinase-catalyzed phosphorylation. Unlike glucose-6-phosphate, however, which is metabolized further eventually to CO_2 and water and to a lesser degree via the hexose-monophosphate shunt, deoxyglucose-6-phosphate cannot be converted to fructose-6-phosphate and is not a substrate for glucose-6-phosphate dehydrogenase. There is very little glucose-6-phosphatase activity in brain and even less deoxyglucose-6-phosphatase activity (Sokoloff and colleagues, 1977). Deoxyglucose-6-phosphate, once formed, is, therefore, essentially trapped in the cerebral tissues, at least long enough for the duration of the measurement.

If the interval of time is kept short enough, for example, less than one hour, to allow the assumption of negligible loss of [14C]DG-6-P from the tissues, then the quantity of [14C]DG-6-P accumulated in any cerebral tissue at any given time following the introduction of [14C]DG into the circulation is equal to the integral of the rate of [14C]DG phosphorylation by hexokinase in that tissue during that interval of time. This integral is in turn related to the amount of glucose that has been phosphorylated over the same interval, depending on the time courses of the relative concentrations of [14C]DG and glucose in the precursor pools and the Michaelis-Menten kinetic constants for hexokinase with respect to both [14C]DG and glucose. With cerebral glucose consumption in a steady state, the amount of glucose phosphorylated during the interval of time equals the steady state flux of glucose through the hexokinase-catalyzed step times the duration of the interval, and the net rate of flux of glucose through this step equals the rate of glucose utilization.

These relationships can be mathematically defined and an operational equation derived if the following assumptions are made: 1) a steady state for glucose (i.e., constant plasma glucose concentration and constant rate of glucose consumption) throughout the period of the procedure; 2) homogeneous tissue compartment within which the concentrations of [14C]DG and glucose are uniform and exchange directly with the plasma; and 3) tracer concentrations of [14C]DG (i.e., molecular concentrations of free [14C]DG essentially equal to zero). The operational equation which defines R_i, the rate of glucose consumption per unit mass of tissue, i, in terms of measurable variables is as follows:

$$R_i = \frac{C_i^* (T) - k_1^* e^{-(k_2^* + k_3^*)T} \int_0^T C_P^* e^{(k_2^* + k_3^*)t} dt}{\left[\dfrac{\lambda V_m^* K_m}{\Phi V_m K_m^*}\right]\left[\int_0^T (C_P^*/C_P) dt - e^{-(k_2^* + k_3^*)T}\int_0^T (C_P^*/C_P) e^{(k_2^* + k_3^*)t} dt\right]} \quad [1]$$

where C_i^* (T) equals the combined concentrations of [14C]DG and [14C]DG-6-P in the tissue, i, at time, T, determined by quantitative autoradiography; C_P^* and C_P equal the arterial plasma concentrations of [14C]DG and glucose, respectively; k_1^*, k_2^*, and k_3^* are the rate constants for the transport from the plasma to the tissue precursor pool, for the transport back from tissue to plasma, and for the phosphorylation of free [14C]DG in the tissue, respectively; λ equals the ratio of the distribution volume of [14C]DG in the tissue to that of glucose; Φ equals the fraction of glucose which once phosphorylated continues down the glycolytic pathway; and K_m^* and V_{max}^* and K_m and V_{max} are the familiar Michaelis-Menten kinetic constants of hexokinase for [14C]DG and glucose, respectively.

The rate constants are determined in a separate group of animals by a non-linear, iterative process which provides the least squares best-fit of an equation which defines the time course of total tissue ^{14}C concentration in terms of the time, the history of the plasma concentration, and the rate constants to the experimentally determined time courses of tissue and plasma concentrations of ^{14}C (Sokoloff and colleagues, 1977). The rate constants have thus far been determined only in the normal conscious albino rat (Sokoloff and colleagues, 1977) and the Rhesus monkey (Kennedy and colleagues, 1978).

The λ, Φ, and the enzyme kinetic constants are grouped together to constitute a single, lumped constant (see equation). It can be shown mathematically that this lumped constant is equal to the asymptotic value of the product of the ratio of the cerebral extraction ratios of [^{14}C]DG and glucose and the ratio of the arterial blood to plasma specific activities when the arterial plasma [^{14}C]DG concentration is maintained constant. The lumped constant is also determined in a separate group of animals from arterial and cerebral venous blood samples drawn during a programmed intravenous infusion which produces and maintains a constant arterial plasma [^{14}C]DG concentration (Sokoloff and colleagues, 1977). Thus far it has been determined only in the rat, monkey, cat, and Beagle puppy (Sokoloff, 1979). The lumped constant appears to be characteristic of the species and does not appear to change significantly in a wide range of conditions (Sokoloff, 1979).

Despite its complex appearance, Equation [1] is really nothing more than a general statement of the standard relationship by which rates of enzyme-catalyzed reactions are determined from measurements made with radioactive tracers. The numerator of the equation represents the amount of radioactive product formed in a given interval of time; it is equal to C_i^*, the combined concentrations of [^{14}C]DG and [^{14}C]DG-6-P in the tissue at time, T, measured by the quantitative autoradiographic technique, less a term that represents the free unmetabolized [^{14}C]DG still remaining in the tissue. The denominator represents the integrated specific activity of the precursor pool times a factor, the lumped constant, which is equivalent to a correction factor for an isotope effect. The term with the exponential factor in the denominator takes into account the lag in the equilibration of the tissue precursor pool with the plasma.

Procedure

Because local rates of cerebral glucose utilization are calculated by means of Equation [1], this equation dictates the variables to be measured. The specific procedure employed is designed to evaluate these variables and to minimize potential errors that might occur in the actual application of the method. If the rate constants, k_1^*, k_2^*, and k_3^*, are precisely known, then Equation [1] is generally applicable with any mode of administration of [^{14}C]DG and for a wide range of time intervals. These rate constants can be expected to vary with the condition of the animal, however, and for most accurate results should be re-determined for each condition studied. The structure of Equation [1] suggests a more practicable alternative. All the terms in the equation that contain the rate constants approach zero with increasing time if the [^{14}C]DG is so administered that the plasma [^{14}C]DG concentration also approaches zero. From the values of the rate constants determined in normal animals and the usual time course of the clearance of [^{14}C]DG from the arterial plasma following a single intravenous pulse at zero time, an interval of 30-45 minutes is adequate for these terms to become sufficiently small that considerable latitude in inaccuracies of the rate constants is permissible without appreciably increased error in the estimates of local glucose consumption (Sokoloff and colleagues, 1977; Sokoloff 1979). An additional advantage derived from the use of a single pulse of [^{14}C]DG followed by a relatively long interval before killing the animal for measurement of local tissue ^{14}C concentration is that by then most of the free [^{14}C]DG in the tissues has been either converted to [^{14}C]DG-6-P or transported back to the plasma; the optical densities in the autoradiographs then represent mainly the concentrations of [^{14}C]DG-6-P and, therefore, reflect directly the relative rates of glucose utilization in the various cerebral tissues.

The experimental procedure is to inject a pulse of [^{14}C]DG intravenously at zero time and to decapitate the animal at a measured time, T, 30-45 minutes later; in the interval timed arterial samples are taken for the measurement of plasma [^{14}C]DG and glucose concentrations. Tissue ^{14}C concentrations, C_i^*, are measured at time, T, by the quantitative autoradiographic technique. Local cerebral glucose utilization is calculated by Equation [1] (Sokoloff and colleagues, 1977).

RATES OF LOCAL CEREBRAL GLUCOSE UTILIZATION IN THE NORMAL CONSCIOUS RAT

Thus far quantitative measurements of local cerebral glucose utilization have been completed only in the albino rat and Rhesus monkey. The values in normal conscious animals are presented in Table 1. The rates of local cerebral glucose utilization in the normal conscious rat vary widely throughout the brain. The values in white structures tend to group together and are always considerably below those of gray structures. The average value in gray matter is approximately 3 times that of white matter, but the individual values vary from approximately 50 to 200 µmoles of glucose/100g/min. The highest values are in the structures involved in auditory functions with the inferior colliculus clearly the most metabolically active structure in the brain.

TABLE 1 Representative Values for Local Cerebral Glucose Utilization in the Normal Conscious Albino Rat and Monkey (µmoles/100g/min)

Structure	*Albino Rat (10)	+Monkey (7)
Gray Matter		
Visual Cortex	107 ± 6	59 ± 2
Auditory Cortex	162 ± 5	79 ± 4
Parietal Cortex	112 ± 5	47 ± 4
Sensory-Motor Cortex	120 ± 5	44 ± 3
Thalamus: Lateral Nucleus	116 ± 5	54 ± 2
Thalamus: Ventral Nucleus	109 ± 5	43 ± 2
Medial Geniculate Body	131 ± 5	65 ± 3
Lateral Geniculate Body	96 ± 5	39 ± 1
Hypothalamus	54 ± 2	25 ± 1
Mamillary Body	121 ± 5	57 ± 3
Hippocampus	79 ± 3	39 ± 2
Amygdala	52 ± 2	25 ± 2
Caudate-Putamen	110 ± 4	52 ± 3
Nucleus Accumbens	82 ± 3	36 ± 2
Globus-Pallidus	58 ± 2	26 ± 2
Substantia Nigra	58 ± 3	29 ± 2
Vestibular Nucleus	128 ± 5	66 ± 3
Cochlear Nucleus	113 ± 7	51 ± 3
Superior Olivary Nucleus	133 ± 7	63 ± 4
Inferior Colliculus	197 ± 10	103 ± 6
Superior Colliculus	95 ± 5	55 ± 4
Pontine Gray Matter	62 ± 3	28 ± 1
Cerebellar Cortex	57 ± 2	31 ± 2
Cerebellar Nuclei	100 ± 4	45 ± 2
White Matter		
Corpus Callosum	40 ± 2	11 ± 1
Internal Capsule	33 ± 2	13 ± 1
Cerebellar White Matter	37 ± 2	12 ± 1

The values are the means ± standard errors from measurements made in the number of animals indicated in parentheses.

* From Sokoloff and colleagues, J. Neurochem. 1977.

+ From Kennedy and colleagues, Annals of Neurol. 1978.

The rates of local cerebral glucose utilization in the normal conscious monkey exhibit similar heterogeneity but they are considerably lower, approximately one-third to one-half those in the rat, probably because of the lower cellular packing density and greater amounts of white matter.

EFFECTS OF GENERAL ANESTHESIA

In the albino rat thiopental anesthesia reduces the rates of glucose utilization in all structures of the brain (Table 2). The effects are not uniform; the percent effects in white matter are relatively small compared to those in most gray structures. Anesthesia also markedly reduces the heterogeneity normally present within gray matter, an effect clearly visible in the autoradiographs (Sokoloff and colleagues, 1977). These results are in agreement with those of previous studies in which anesthesia has been found to decrease the cerebral metabolic rate of the brain as a whole (Kety, 1950; Lassen, 1959; Sokoloff, 1976).

TABLE 2   Effects of Thiopental Anesthesia on Local Cerebral
Glucose Utilization in the Rat * §

Structure	Local Cerebral Glucose Utilization (µmoles/100g/min)		% Effect
	Control (6)†	Anesthetized (8)†	
Gray Matter			
Visual Cortex	111 ± 5	64 ± 3	− 42
Auditory Cortex	157 ± 5	81 ± 3	− 48
Parietal Cortex	107 ± 3	65 ± 2	− 39
Sensory-Motor Cortex	118 ± 3	67 ± 2	− 43
Lateral Geniculate Body	92 ± 2	53 ± 3	− 42
Medial Geniculate Body	126 ± 6	63 ± 3	− 50
Thalamus: Lateral Nucleus	108 ± 3	58 ± 2	− 46
Thalamus: Ventral Nucleus	98 ± 3	55 ± 1	− 44
Hypothalamus	63 ± 3	43 ± 2	− 32
Caudate-Putamen	111 ± 4	72 ± 3	− 35
Hippocampus: Ammon's Horn	79 ± 1	56 ± 1	− 29
Amygdala	56 ± 4	41 ± 2	− 27
Cochlear Nucleus	124 ± 7	79 ± 5	− 36
Lateral Lemniscus	114 ± 7	75 ± 4	− 34
Inferior Colliculus	198 ± 7	131 ± 8	− 34
Superior Olivary Nucleus	141 ± 5	104 ± 7	− 26
Superior Colliculus	99 ± 3	59 ± 3	− 40
Vestibular Nucleus	133 ± 4	81 ± 4	− 39
Pontine Gray Matter	69 ± 3	46 ± 3	− 33
Cerebellar Cortex	66 ± 2	44 ± 2	− 33
Cerebellar Nucleus	106 ± 4	75 ± 4	− 29
White Matter			
Corpus Callosum	42 ± 2	30 ± 2	− 29
Genu of Corpus Callosum	35 ± 5	30 ± 2	− 14
Internal Capsule	35 ± 2	29 ± 2	− 17
Cerebellar White Matter	38 ± 2	29 ± 2	− 24

* Determined at 30 minutes following pulse of [^{14}C]deoxyglucose.

† The values are the means ± standard errors obtained in the number of animals indicated in parentheses. All the differences are statistically significant at the $p < 0.05$ level.

§ From Sokoloff and colleagues (1977).

RELATION BETWEEN LOCAL FUNCTIONAL ACTIVITY AND ENERGY METABOLISM

The results of a variety of applications of the method demonstrate a clear relationship between local cerebral functional activity and glucose consumption. The most striking demonstrations of the close coupling between function and energy metabolism are seen with experimentally induced local alterations in functional activity that are restricted to a few specific areas in the brain. The effects on local glucose consumption are then so pronounced that they are not only observed in the quantitative results but can be visualized directly on the autoradiographs which are really pictorial representations of the relative rates of glucose utilization in the various structural components of the brain.

Effects of Increased Functional Activity

Effects of sciatic nerve stimulation. Electrical stimulation of one sciatic nerve
in the rat under barbiturate anesthesia causes pronounced increases in glucose
consumption (i.e., increased optical density in the autoradiographs) in the ipsilateral dorsal horn of the lumbar spinal cord (Kennedy and colleagues, 1975).

Effects of experimental focal seizures. The local injection of penicillin into the
hand-face area of the motor cortex of the rhesus monkey has been shown to induce
electrical discharges in the adjacent cortex and to result in recurrent focal
seizures involving the face, arm, and hand on the contralateral side (Caveness,
1969). Such seizure activity causes selective increases in glucose consumption in
areas of motor cortex adjacent to the penicillin locus and in small discrete regions
of the putamen, globus pallidus, caudate nucleus, thalamus, and substantia nigra of
the same side (Fig. 1) (Kennedy and colleagues, 1975). Similar studies in the rat
have led to comparable results and provided evidence on the basis of an evoked
metabolic response of a "mirror" focus in the motor cortex contralateral to the
penicillin-induced epileptogenic focus (Collins and colleagues, 1976).

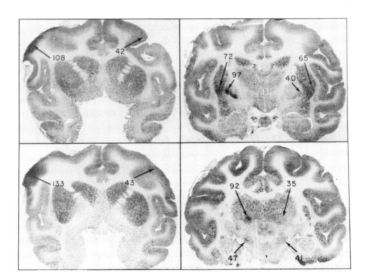

Fig. 1.   Effects of focal seizures produced by local application of penicillin to
motor cortex on local cerebral glucose utilization in the rhesus monkey. The
penicillin was applied to the hand and face area of the left motor cortex. The
left side of the brain is on the left in each of the autoradiographs in the figure.
The numbers are the rates of local cerebral glucose utilization in μmoles/100 g
tissue/min. Note the following: Upper left, motor cortex in region of penicillin
application and corresponding region of contralateral motor cortex; Lower left,
ipsilateral and contralateral motor cortical regions remote from area of penicillin
applications; Upper right, ipsilateral and contralateral putamen and globus pallidus;
Lower right, ipsilateral and contralateral thalamic nuclei and substantia nigra.
From Kennedy and colleagues (1975).

Effects of Decreased Functional Activity

Decrements in functional activity result in reduced rates of glucose utilization.
These effects are particularly striking in the auditory and visual systems of the
rat and the visual system of the monkey.

Effects of auditory deprivation.   In the albino rat some of the highest rates of
local cerebral glucose utilization are found in components of the auditory system,
i.e., auditory cortex, medial geniculate ganglion, inferior colliculus, lateral
lemniscus, superior olive, and cochlear nucleus (Table 1).   The high metabolic
activities of some of these structures are clearly visible in the autoradiographs
(Fig. 2).   Bilateral auditory deprivation by occlusion of both external auditory
canals with wax markedly depresses the metabolic activity in all of these areas
(Fig. 2) (Des Rosiers, Kennedy and Sokoloff, unpublished observations).   The reductions are symmetrical bilaterally and range from 35 to 60 percent.   Unilateral
auditory deprivation also depresses the glucose consumption of these structures
but to a lesser degree, and some of the structures are asymmetrically affected.
For example, the metabolic activity of the ipsilateral cochlear nucleus equals 75
percent of the activity of the contralateral nucleus.   The lateral lemniscus,
superior olive, and medial geniculate ganglion are slightly lower on the contralateral side while the contralateral inferior colliculus is markedly lower in
metabolic activity than the ipsilateral structure (Fig. 2).   These results
demonstrate that there is some degree of lateralization and crossing of auditory
pathways in the rat.

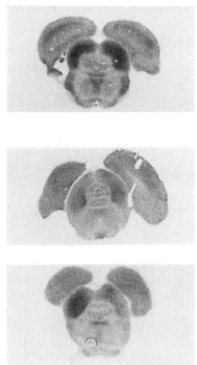

Fig. 2.   Effects of auditory deprivation on cerebral glucose utilization of some
components of the auditory system of the albino rat.   Upper, autoradiograph of
section of brain from normal conscious rat with intact bilateral hearing in ambient
noise of laboratory.   The autoradiograph shows the inferior colliculi, the lateral

lemnisci, and the superior olives, all of which exhibit bilateral symmetry of optical densities. Middle, autoradiograph of comparable section of brain from rat with bilateral occlusion of external auditory canals with wax and kept in sound-proof room. Note the virtual disappearance of the inferior colliculi, lateral lemnisci, and superior olives. Lower, autoradiograph of comparable section of brain from rat with one external auditory canal blocked. Note the asymmetry of the inferior colliculi, and the almost symmetrical intermediate reductions of densities in the lateral lemnisci and superior olives. The ear that was blocked was contra-lateral to the inferior colliculus that was markedly depressed. From Des Rosiers, Kennedy, and Sokoloff (unpublished observations).

Visual deprivation in the rat. In the rat, the visual system is 80 to 85 percent crossed at the optic chiasma (Lashley, 1934; Montero and Guillery, 1968), and unilateral enucleation removes most of the visual input to the central visual structures of the contralateral side. In the conscious rat studied 24 hours after unilateral enucleation, there are marked decrements in glucose utilization in the contralateral superior colliculus, lateral geniculate ganglion, and visual cortex as compared to the ipsilateral side (Fig. 3) (Kennedy and colleagues, 1975). In the rat with both eyes intact, no asymmetry in the autoradiographs is observed (Fig. 3).

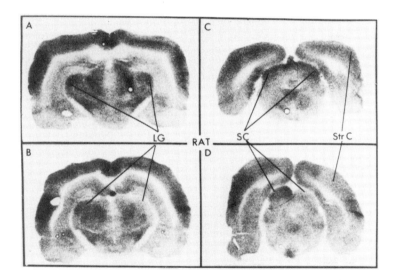

Fig. 3.   Effects of unilateral enucleation on [^{14}C]deoxyglucose uptake in components of the visual system in the rat. In the normal rat with both eyes intact the uptakes in the lateral geniculate bodies (LG), superior colliculi (SC) and striate cortex (STR C) are approximately equal on both sides (A and C). In the unilaterally enucleated rat there are marked decreases in optical densities in the areas corres-ponding to these structures on the side contralateral to the enucleation (B and D). From Kennedy and colleagues (1975).

<u>Visual deprivation in the monkey</u>. In animals with binocular visual systems, such
as the Rhesus monkey, there is only approximately 50 percent crossing of the visual
pathways, and the structures of the visual system on each side of the brain receive
equal inputs from both retinae. Although each retina projects more or less equally
to both hemispheres, their projections remain segregated and terminate in six well-
defined laminae in the lateral geniculate ganglia, three each for the ipsilateral
and contralateral eyes (Hubel and Wiesel, 1968, 1972; Wiesel and colleagues, 1974;
Rakic, 1976). This segregation is preserved in the optic radiations which project
the monocular representations of the two eyes for any segment of the visual field
to adjacent regions of Layer IV of the striate cortex (Hubel and Wiesel, 1968,
1972). The cells responding to the input of each monocular terminal zone are
distributed transversely through the thickness of the striate cortex resulting in
a mosaic of columns, 0.3-0.5 mm in width, alternately representing the monocular
inputs of the two eyes. The nature and distribution of these ocular dominance
columns have previously been characterized by electrophysiological techniques
(Hubel and Wiesel, 1968), Nauta degeneration methods (Hubel and Wiesel, 1972),
and by autoradiographic visualization of axonal and transneuronal transport of
[^{3}H]proline- and [^{3}H]fucose-labeled protein and/or glycoprotein (Wiesel and
colleagues, 1974; Rakic, 1976). Bilateral or unilateral visual deprivation, either
by enucleation or by the insertion of opaque plastic discs, produce consistent
changes in the pattern of distribution of the rates of glucose consumption, all
clearly visible in the autoradiographs, that coincide closely with the changes in
functional activity expected from known physiological and anatomic properties of
the binocular visual system (Kennedy and colleagues, 1976).

In animals with intact binocular vision no bilateral asymmetry is seen in the
autoradiographs of the structures of the visual system (Figs. 4A, 5A). The lateral
geniculate ganglia and oculomotor nuclei appear to be of fairly uniform density and
essentially the same on both sides (Fig. 4A). The visual cortex is also the same
on both sides (Fig. 5A), but throughout all of Area 17 there is heterogeneous
density distributed in a characteristic laminar pattern. These observations indicate that in animals with binocular visual input the rates of glucose consumption
in the visual pathways are essentially equal on both sides of the brain and relatively uniform in the oculomotor nuclei and lateral geniculate ganglia, but markedly different in the various layers of the striate cortex.

Autoradiographs from animals with both eyes occluded exhibit generally decreased
labeling of all components of the visual system, but the bilateral symmetry is
fully retained (Figs. 4B, 5B), and the density within each lateral geniculate body
is for the most part fairly uniform (Fig. 4B). In the striate cortex, however, the
marked differences in the densities of the various layers seen in the animals with
intact bilateral vision (Fig. 5A) are virtually absent so that, except for a faint
delineation of a band within Layer IV, the concentration of the label is essentially
homogeneous throughout the striate cortex (Fig. 5B).

Autoradiographs from monkeys with only monocular input because of unilateral visual
occlusion exhibit markedly different patterns from those described above. Both
lateral geniculate bodies exhibit exactly inverse patterns of alternating dark and
light bands corresponding to the known laminae representing the regions receiving
the different inputs from the retinae of the intact and occluded eyes (Fig. 4C).
Bilateral asymmetry is also seen in the oculomotor nuclear complex; a lower density
is apparent in the nuclear complex contralateral to the occluded eye (Fig. 4C). In
the striate cortex the pattern of distribution of the [^{14}C]DG-6-P appears to be a
composite of the patterns seen in the animals with intact and bilaterally occluded
visual input. The pattern found in the former regularly alternates with that of
the latter in columns oriented perpendicularly to the cortical surface (Fig. 5C).
The dimensions, arrangement, and distribution of these columns are identical to
those of the ocular dominance columns described by Hubel and Wiesel (Hubel and

Wiesel, 1968, 1972; Wiesel and colleagues, 1974). These columns reflect the inter-
digitation of the representations of the two retinae in the visual cortex. Each
element in the visual fields is represented by a pair of contiguous bands in the
visual cortex, one for each of the two retinae or their portions that correspond to
the given point in the visual fields. With symmetrical visual input bilaterally,
the columns representing the two eyes are equally active and, therefore, not
visualized in the autoradiographs (Fig. 5A). When one eye is blocked, however,
only those columns representing the blocked eye become metabolically less active,
and the autoradiographs then display the alternate bands of normal and depressed
activities corresponding to the regions of visual cortical representation of the
two eyes (Fig. 5C).

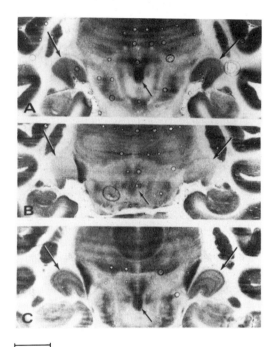

5.0mm

Fig. 4.   Autoradiographs of coronal brain sections from Rhesus monkeys at the
level of the lateral geniculate bodies. Large arrows point to the lateral geniculate bodies; small arrows point to oculomotor nuclear complex. A) Animal with
intact binocular vision. Note the bilateral symmetry and relative homogeneity of
the lateral geniculate bodies and oculomotor nuclei. B) Animal with bilateral
visual occlusion. Note the reduced relative densities, the relative homogeneity,
and the bilateral symmetry of the lateral geniculate bodies and oculomotor nuclei.
C) Animal with right eye occluded. The left side of the brain is on the left side
of the photograph. Note the laminae and the inverse order of the dark and light
bands in the two lateral geniculate bodies. Note also the lesser density of the
oculomotor nuclear complex on the side contralateral to the occluded eye. From
Kennedy and colleagues (1976).

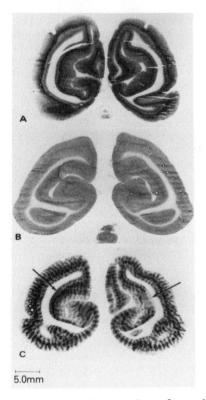

5.0mm

Fig. 5.   Autoradiographs of coronal brain sections from rhesus monkeys at the
level of the striate cortex. A) Animal with normal binocular vision. Note the
laminar distribution of the density; the dark band corresponds to Layer IV.
B) Animal with bilateral visual deprivation. Note the almost uniform and reduced
relative density, especially the virtual disappearance of the dark band corresponding to Layer IV. C) Animal with right eye occluded. The half-brain on the
left side of the photograph represents the left hemisphere contralateral to the
occluded eye. Note the alternate dark and light striations, each approximately
0.3-0.4 mm in width, representing the ocular dominance columns. These columns are
most apparent in the dark lamina corresponding to Layer IV but extend through the
entire thickness of the cortex. The arrows point to regions of bilateral asymmetry
where the ocular dominance columns are absent. These are presumably areas with
normally only monocular input. The one on left, contralateral to occluded eye, has
a continuous dark lamina corresponding to Layer IV which is completely absent on
the side ipsilateral to the occluded eye. These regions are believed to be the
loci of the cortical representations of the blind spots. From Kennedy and colleagues
(1976).

There can be seen in the autoradiographs from the animals with unilateral visual
deprivation a pair of regions in the folded calcarine cortex that exhibit bilateral
asymmetry (Fig. 5C). The ocular dominance columns are absent on both sides, but on
the side contralateral to the occluded eye this region has the appearance of visual
cortex from an animal with normal bilateral vision, and on the ipsilateral side this
region looks like cortex from an animal with both eyes occluded (Fig. 5). These
regions are the loci of the cortical representation of the blind spots of the visual
fields and normally have only monocular input (Kennedy and colleagues, 1975, 1976).
The area of the optic disc in the nasal half of each retina cannot transmit to this

region of the contralateral striate cortex which, therefore, receives its sole input from an area in the temporal half of the ipsilateral retina. Occlusion of one eye deprives this region of the ipsilateral striate cortex of all input while the corresponding region of the contralateral striate cortex retains uninterrupted input from the intact eye. The metabolic reflection of this ipsilateral monocular input is seen in the autoradiograph in Fig. 5C.

The results of these studies with the [^{14}C]deoxyglucose method in the binocular visual system of the monkey represent the most dramatic demonstration of the close relationship between physiological changes in functional activity and the rate of energy metabolism in specific components of the central nervous system.

Pharmacological Studies

The ability of the [^{14}C]deoxyglucose method to map the entire brain for localized regions of altered functional activity on the basis of changes in energy metabolism offers a potent tool to identify the neural sites of action of agents with neuro-pharmacological and psychopharmacological actions.

Effects of carbon dioxide. The inhalation of 5 to 10 percent CO_2, which increases cerebral blood flow and produces desynchronization and a shift to higher frequency activity in the electroencephalogram, causes in the conscious rat moderate but diffuse reductions in local cerebral glucose utilization (Des Rosiers and colleagues, 1976).

Effects of γ-hydroxybutyrate. γ-Hydroxybutyrate and γ-butyrolactone, which is hydrolyzed to γ-hydroxybutyrate in plasma, produce trance-like behavioral states associated with marked suppression of electroencephalographic activity (Giarman and Roth, 1964). These effects are reversible, and these drugs have been used clinically as anesthetic adjuvants. There is evidence that these agents lower neuronal activity in the nigrostriatal pathway and may act by inhibition of dopa-minergic synapses (Roth, 1976). Studies in rats with the [^{14}C]deoxyglucose technique have demonstrated that γ-butyrolactone produces profound dose-dependent reductions of glucose utilization throughout the brain (Wolfson and colleagues, 1976). At the highest doses studied, 600 mg per kg of body weight, glucose utilization was reduced by approximately 75 percent in gray matter and 33 percent in white matter, but there was no obvious further specificity with respect to the local cerebral structures affected. The reversibility of the effects and the magnitude and diffuseness of the depression of cerebral metabolic rate suggests that this drug might be considered as a chemical substitute for hypothermia in conditions in which profound reversible reduction of cerebral metabolism is desired.

Effects of amphetamines. Enhancement of dopaminergic synaptic activity by admini-stration of d-amphetamine (Wechsler, Savaki and Sokoloff, 1979), which stimulates release of dopamine at the synapse, produces marked increases in glucose con-sumption in all the components of the extrapyramidal system known or suspected to contain dopamine-receptive cells (Table 3). The greatest increases noted were in the zona reticulata of the substantia nigra and the subthalamic nucleus. Reduc-tions were noted in the suprachiasmatic nucleus of the hypothalamus and the habenula. l-Amphetamine exhibited markedly lesser effects.

L. Sokoloff

TABLE 3   Effects of d-Amphetamine and l-Amphetamine on
Local Cerebral Glucose Utilization in the Conscious Rat +

	control	d-amphetamine	l-amphetamine
Gray Matter			
Visual Cortex	102 ± 8	135 ± 11*	105 ± 8
Auditory Cortex	160 ± 11	162 ± 6	141 ± 6
Parietal Cortex	109 ± 9	125 ± 10	116 ± 4
Sensory-Motor Cortex	118 ± 8	139 ± 9	111 ± 4
Olfactory Cortex	100 ± 6	93 ± 5	94 ± 3
Frontal Cortex	109 ± 10	130 ± 8	105 ± 4
Prefrontal Cortex	146 ± 10	166 ± 7	154 ± 4
Thalamus - Lateral Nucleus	97 ± 5	114 ± 8	117 ± 6
- Ventral Nucleus	85 ± 7	108 ± 6*	96 ± 4
- Habenula	118 ± 10	71 ± 5**	82 ± 2**
- Dorsomedial Nucleus	92 ± 6	111 ± 8	106 ± 6
Medial Geniculate	116 ± 5	119 ± 4	116 ± 4
Lateral Geniculate	79 ± 5	88 ± 5	84 ± 4
Hypothalamus	54 ± 5	56 ± 3	52 ± 3
- Suprachiasmatic Nucleus	94 ± 4	75 ± 4**	67 ± 1**
- Mamillary Body	117 ± 8	134 ± 5	142 ± 5*
Lateral Olfactory Nucleus§	92 ± 6	95 ± 5	99 ± 6
A_{13}	71 ± 4	91 ± 4**	81 ± 4
Hippocampus - Ammon's Horn	79 ± 5	73 ± 2	81 ± 6
- Dentate Gyrus	60 ± 4	55 ± 3	67 ± 7
Amygdala	46 ± 3	46 ± 3	44 ± 2
Septal Nucleus	56 ± 3	55 ± 2	54 ± 3
Caudate Nucleus	109 ± 5	132 ± 8*	127 ± 3*
Nucleus Accumbens	76 ± 5	80 ± 3	78 ± 3
Globus Pallidus	53 ± 3	64 ± 2*	65 ± 3*
Subthalamic Nucleus	89 ± 6	149 ± 10**	107 ± 2
Substantia Nigra - Zona Reticulata	58 ± 2	105 ± 4**	72 ± 4
- Zona Compacta	65 ± 4	88 ± 6**	72 ± 3
Red Nucleus	76 ± 5	94 ± 5*	86 ± 2
Vestibular Nucleus	121 ± 11	137 ± 5	130 ± 4
Cochlear Nucleus	139 ± 6	126 ± 1	141 ± 5
Superior Olivary Nucleus	144 ± 4	143 ± 4	147 ± 6
Lateral Lemniscus	107 ± 3	96 ± 5	98 ± 3
Inferior Colliculus	193 ± 10	169 ± 5	150 ± 8**
Dorsal Tegmental Nucleus	109 ± 5	112 ± 7	122 ± 6
Superior Colliculus	80 ± 5	89 ± 3	91 ± 3
Pontine Gray	58 ± 4	65 ± 3	60 ± 1
Cerebellar Flocculus	124 ± 10	146 ± 15	153 ± 10
Cerebellar Hemispheres	55 ± 3	68 ± 6	64 ± 2
Cerebellar Nuclei	102 ± 4	105 ± 8	110 ± 3
White Matter			
Corpus Callosum	23 ± 3	24 ± 2	23 ± 1
Genu of Corpus Callosum	29 ± 2	30 ± 2	26 ± 2
Internal Capsule	21 ± 1	24 ± 2	19 ± 2
Cerebellar White	28 ± 1	31 ± 2	31 ± 2

+ All values are the means ± standard error of the mean for five animals.
* Significant difference from the control at the $p < 0.05$ level.
** Significant difference from the control at the $p < 0.01$ level.
§ It was not possible to correlate precisely this area on autoradiographs with a
  specific structure in the rat brain. It is, however, most likely the lateral
  olfactory nucleus.
From Wechsler, Savaki, and Sokoloff (1979)

Effects of LSD. The effects of the potent psychotomimetic agent, D-lysergic acid
diethylamide, have been examined in the rat (Shinohara and colleagues, 1976). In
doses of 12.5 to 125 µg/kg, it caused dose-dependent reductions in glucose utilization in a number of cerebral structures. With increasing dosage more structures
were affected and to a greater degree. There was no pattern in the distribution of
the effects, at least none discernible at the present level of resolution, that
might contribute to the understanding of the drug's psychotomimetic actions.

Effects of morphine addiction and withdrawal. Acute morphine administration
depresses glucose utilization in many areas of the brain, but the specific effects
of morphine could not be distinguished from those of the hypercapnia produced by
the associated respiratory depression (Sakurada and colleagues, 1976). In contrast,
morphine addiction, produced within 24 hours by a single subcutaneous injection of
150 mg/kg of morphine base in an oil emulsion, reduces glucose utilization in a
large number of gray structures in the absence of changes in arterial pCO_2. White
matter appears to be unaffected. Naloxone (one mg/kg subcutaneously) reduces
glucose utilization in a number of structures when administered to normal rats, but
when given to the morphine-addicted animals produces an acute withdrawal-syndrome
and reverses the reductions of glucose utilization in several of the structures,
most strikingly in the habenula (Sakurada and colleagues, 1976).

SUMMARY

The results of studies with the [14C]deoxyglucose technique unequivocally establish
that functional activity in specific components of the central nervous system is,
as in other tissues, closely coupled to the local rate of energy metabolism.

Stimulation of functional activity increases the local rate of glucose utilization; reduced functional activity depresses it. These changes are so profound that they can be visualized directly in autoradiographic representations of local tissue concentrations of [^{14}C]deoxyglucose-6-phosphate. Indeed, the existence of such evoked metabolic responses to experimentally induced alterations in local functional activity, together with the ability to visualize them by the [^{14}C]deoxyglucose method, has become the basis of a potent technique for the mapping of functional pathways in the central nervous system (Kennedy and colleagues, 1975, 1976; Plum and colleagues, 1976).

REFERENCES

Caveness, W. F. (1969). Ontogeny of focal seizures. In H. H. Jasper, A. A. Ward, and A. Pope (Eds.), Basic Mechanisms of the Epilepsies. Little, Brown and Co., Boston. pp. 517-534.

Collins, R. C., C. Kennedy, L. Sokoloff, and F. Plum (1976). Metabolic anatomy of focal seizures. Arch. Neurol., 33, 536-542.

Des Rosiers, M. H., C. Kennedy, M. Shinohara, and L. Sokoloff (1976). Effects of CO_2 on local cerebral glucose utilization in the conscious rat. Neurology, 26(4), 346.

Giarman, N. J. and R. H. Roth (1964). Differential estimation of γ-butyrolactone and γ-hydroxybutyric acid in rat blood and brain. Science, 145, 583-584.

Hubel, D. H. and T. N. Wiesel (1968). Receptive fields and functional architecture of monkey striate cortex. J. Physiol., 195, 215-243.

Hubel, D. H. and T. N. Wiesel (1972). Laminar and columnar distribution of geniculo-cortical fibers in the Macaque monkey. J. Comp. Neurol., 146, 421-450.

Kennedy, C., M. H. Des Rosiers, M. Reivich, F. Sharp, J. W. Jehle, and L. Sokoloff (1975). Mapping of functional neural pathways by autoradiographic survey of local metabolic rate with [^{14}C]deoxyglucose. Science, 187, 850-853.

Kennedy, C., M. H. Des Rosiers, O. Sakurada, M. Shinohara, M. Reivich, J. W. Jehle, and L. Sokoloff (1976). Metabolic mapping of the primary visual system of the monkey by means of the autoradiographic [^{14}C]deoxyglucose technique. Proc. Natl. Acad. Sci. USA, 73, 4230-4234.

Kennedy, C., O. Sakurada, M. Shinohara, J. Jehle, and L. Sokoloff (1978). Local cerebral glucose utilization in the normal conscious Macaque monkey. Ann. Neurol., 4, 293-301.

Kety, S. S. (1950). Circulation and metabolism of the human brain in health and disease. Amer. J. Med., 8, 205-217.

Kety, S. S. (1957). The general metabolism of the brain in vivo. In D. Richter (Ed.), The Metabolism of the Nervous System. Pergamon Press, London. pp. 221-237.

Landau, W. M., W. H. Freygang, L. P. Rowland, L. Sokoloff, and S. S. Kety (1955). The local circulation of the living brain; values in the unanesthetized and anesthetized cat. Trans. Am. Neurol. Assoc., 80, 125-129.

Lashley, K. S. (1934). The mechanism of vision. VII. The projection of the retina upon the primary optic centers of the rat. J. Comp. Neurol., 59, 341-373.

Lassen, N. A. (1959). Cerebral blood flow and oxygen consumption in man. Physiol. Rev., 39, 183-238.

Montero, V. M. and R. W. Guillery (1968). Degeneration in the dorsal lateral geniculate nucleus of the rat following interruption of the retinal or cortical connections. J. Comp. Neurol., 134, 211-242.

Plum, F., A. Gjedde, and F. E. Samson (Eds.) (1976). Neuroanatomical functional mapping by the radioactive 2-deoxy-D-glucose method. Neurosci. Res. Program Bull., 14, 457-518.

Rakic, P. (1976). Prenatal genesis of connections subserving ocular dominance in the Rhesus monkey. Nature, 261, 467-471.

Reivich, M., J. W. Jehle, L. Sokoloff, and S. S. Kety (1969). Measurement of
     regional cerebral blood flow with antipyrine-C^{14} in awake cats. J. Appl.
     Physiol., 27, 296-300.
Roth, R. H. (1976). Striatal dopamine and gamma-hydroxybutyrate. Pharmac. and
     Ther., 2, 71-88.
Sakurada, O., M. Shinohara, W. A. Klee, C. Kennedy, and L. Sokoloff (1976). Neuro-
     science Abstr., 2 (Part 1), 613.
Sharp, F. R., J. S. Kauer, and G. M. Shepherd (1975). Local sites of activity-
     related glucose metabolism in rat olfactory bulb during olfactory stimulation.
     Brain Res., 98, 596-600.
Shinohara, M., O. Sakurada, J. Jehle, and L. Sokoloff (1976). Effects of D-lysergic
     acid diethylamide on local cerebral glucose utilization in the rat. Neurosci.
     Abstr., 2 (Part 1), 615.
Sokoloff, L. (1969). Cerebral circulation and behavior in man: strategy and find-
     ings. In A. J. Mandell and M. P. Mandell (Eds.), Psychochemical Research in
     Man. Academic Press, New York City. pp. 237-252.
Sokoloff, L. (1976). Circulation and energy metabolism of the brain. In G. J.
     Siegel, R. W. Albers, R. Katzman, and B. W. Agranoff (Eds.), Basic Neuro-
     chemistry, Second Edition. Little, Brown and Co., Boston. pp. 388-413.
Sokoloff, L., M. Reivich, C. Kennedy, M. H. Des Rosiers, C. S. Patlak, K. D.
     Pettigrew, O. Sakurada, and M. Shinohara (1977). The [^{14}C]deoxyglucose method
     for the measurement of local cerebral glucose utilization: theory, procedure,
     and normal values in the conscious and anesthetized albino rat. J. Neurochem.,
     28, 897-916.
Sokoloff, L. (1979). The [^{14}C]deoxyglucose method: four years later. In F. Gotoh,
     H. Nagai, and Y. Tazaki (Eds.), Cerebral Blood Flow and Metabolism. Munksgard,
     Copenhagen. pp. 640-649.
Wechsler, L. R., H. E. Savaki, and L. Sokoloff (1979). Effects of d- and l-ampheta-
     mine on local cerebral glucose utilization in the conscious rat. J. Neurochem.,
     32, 15-22.
Wiesel, T. N., D. H. Hubel, and D. M. K. Lam (1974). Autoradiographic demonstra-
     tion of ocular dominance columns in the monkey striate cortex by means of
     transneuronal transport. Brain Res., 79, 273-279.
Wolfson, L. I., O. Sakurada, and L. Sokoloff (1976). Effects of γ-hydroxybutyrate
     on local cerebral glucose utilization. Trans. Am. Soc. Neurochem., 7, 165.

DISCUSSION

Mandel: Thank you Dr. Sokoloff for your extremely interesting topic. Now let us start discussion because time is largely over. Questions or comments?

Hudlicka: The results are really fascinating. I would like to ask you whether you made any attempts to put your data together with those of Prof. Lassen from Copenhaguen who is using the Xenon clearance technique to measure blood flow in different parts of the brain.

Sokoloff: He measures blood flow, not energy metabolism. He measures only in the cerebral cortex and in man. Therefore it's difficult to relate our data to his. We have compared blood flow and metabolism in animals, in the rat, and there the correlation is very good. You know that we have another method for measuring local cerebral blood flow that also uses autoradiography. This method uses carbon-14-labelled-iodoantipyrine, and it's possible to measure the rates of blood flow in the same structures where we measured the rates of utilization of glucose. In this slide are represented four groups of animals: in one group we measured blood flow by this method and in the other, we measured glucose utilization, both measurements in conscious animals. We also repeated similar studies in anesthetized animals. Each point here represents the mean of 8 animals in each group for a specific structure. The correlation between blood flow and metabolism is extremely good in the conscious animals; the correlation coefficient is 0.95. In anesthetized animals, the metabolism is lower, in general, blood flow is too. The correlation still remains pretty good, but not nearly as good as in the conscious animals, because the blood flow responds to changes in blood pH, blood pCO_2 etc., factors not directly related to cerebral energy metabolism. If anything alters the blood composition in a way that affects blood flow independently, then the correlation with metabolism will be inpaired.

Porsche: Could deoxyglucose influence the glycogenogenetic pathway?

Sokoloff: No, it does not get into glycogen. The deoxyglucose-6-phosphate can not be metabolized by the glycolytic pathway.

Hoyer: Well, I think that this method is of great importance and validity, especially in the investigation of patients. And my question concerns patients: is the application of deoxyglucose performed as a bolus injection or as an infusion? If the latter was used, then the question arises whether the competition between glucose and deoxyglucose can change energy metabolism.

Sokoloff: It is given as a bolus over a very short time, and we keep the dose sufficiently low so that there is no chance that we will have a pharmacological effect.

Hossmann: Dr. Sokoloff, is it possible to use this technique in pathological states, particularly under hypoxic and ischemic conditions? I see two problems: One is the problem of the different rate constants, and the other problem is the low yield of glucose metabolism under anaerobic conditions. Glucose utilization therefore does not longer parallel the energy production of the tissue.

Sokoloff: In all cases, we measure glucose utilization. The method does not distinguish whether the glucose is being metabolized only to lactate or whether

it's going all the way to CO_2 and H_2O. Now, if lactate is accumulating, obviously glucose utilization and overall energy metabolism are not the same. That's why we say that glucose utilization is a measure of overall energy metabolism only in a steady state. Now, for the questions about the pathological conditions: It is likely that one will have to redetermine lumped constant for pathological con-ditions. It's absolutely sure, but one can think of reasons why it might change. We do know now that the lumped constant does change in severe hypoglycemia and severe hyperglycemia, and so since we want to study these conditions, we have just now determined lumped constants for those conditions. The rate constants are not nearly as much of a problem. If the rate constants were to change in a direction in which they get bigger, it will not make much difference. If they get very much lower, then they might be a problem, but they can be redetermined, too.
We are now in the process to redetermine them in hypoglycemia and hyperglycemia. Ischemia is another problem. In fact, I don't quite understand why you would like to measure glucose utilization in ischemia. The reason that you have a patholo-gical state then is because there is not enough nutritive material brought to tissue. Then we know that the glucose utilization has to be reduced, if there is not enough being brought. During recovery from ischemia, that's another matter. When you restore the blood flow and restore the substrate supply, you might want to know whether the tissues can use it. Then you can probably use the method without redetermining lumped constant.

Energy Metabolism in Isolated Rat Brain

J. Krieglstein, B. Dirks and J. Hanke

Institut für Pharmakologie und Toxikologie, Fachbereich
Pharmazie und Lebensmittelchemie der Philipps-Universität,
Ketzerbach 63, D-3550 Marburg (Lahn),
Federal Republic of Germany

ABSTRACT

An isolated perfused rat brain preparation was proposed for investigations on brain energy metabolism. A perfusion medium containing a
fluorocarbon as an oxygen carrier was successfully used. The spontaneous EEG of the isolated rat brain proved to be a sensitive criterion
of brain viability. Drugs produced specific and dose-dependent EEG
changes. The energy state of the isolated rat brain was similar to
that of rat brain in vivo. It was possible to maintain the isolated
rat brain for several hours with spontaneous EEG activity and without
histological evidence of damage. Ischemia was achieved by interrupting
the flow to the isolated rat brain for 1 min. The EEG disappeared
within 30 sec and reappeared when the circulation was resumed.
Ischemia accelerated glycolysis and significantly reduced the adenylate energy charge. The barbiturate methohexital retards these changes
in energy metabolism. It was pointed out that the clear-cut experimental conditions of the isolated perfused rat brain may be particularly useful for studies on energy metabolism.

KEYWORDS

Isolated perfused rat brain; energy metabolism; EEG; ischemia;
glycolysis; high-energy phosphates; methohexital.

INTRODUCTION

Brain energy metabolism has widely been examined in vivo with laboratory animals or in vitro with tissue slices, cellular particles or
enzymes. An isolated brain preparation, however, offers essential
advantages since this procedure maintains anatomical integrity of the
organ while permitting an absolute control of the arterial supply to
the brain. In addition, the activity of the brain is not affected by
secondary peripheral actions such as liver or muscle metabolism,
cardiovascular or respiratory effects.

A number of different animal species have been used for isolated brain
perfusion (for a review, see Krieglstein and Stock, 1974; Woods and

Youdim, 1977). The rat is favoured for this technique because of ease
of preparation and low cost. Furthermore, the wide-spread use of this
animal for brain research also enables scientists to compare the results obtained from isolated rat brain with those from other preparations using the rat. The isolated perfused rat brain according to
Andjus et al. (1967) as standardized in our laboratory (Krieglstein et
al., 1972a; 1972b; Dirks et al., 1980) is capable of maintaining a
normal energy metabolism, spontaneous electrical activity and vascular
resistance for several hours. Thus, this preparation seems to be
appropriate for investigations on cerebral metabolism.

MATERIALS AND METHODS

Materials. The enzymes, coenzymes and substrates were purchased from
Boehringer, Mannheim. Bovine serum albumin was obtained from Behring-
werke, Marburg (quality: pure, dry). The fluorocarbon FC 43[R] (perfluorotributylamine) was purchased from 3M Company (Neuss), Pluronic F
68 (high molecular weight block polymer of oxyethylene and oxypropyl-
ene) from BASF Wyandotte (Erbslöh, Düsseldorf). All other chemicals
were of reagent grade.

Experimental animals. Male Sprague-Dawley or Wistar rats, weighing
180 - 250 g, were kept on a standard diet (Altromin[R], Lage/Lippe)
and tap water ad libitum.

Perfusion technique. The method of brain perfusion used is based on
the procedure of Andjus et al. (1967), as modified and standardized
in our laboratory (Krieglstein et al., 1972a, 1972b; Dirks et al.,
1980). In order to prepare them, the rats were anesthetized by intraperitoneal injection of 1.2 g/kg urethan. A perfusion apparatus with
one or two circuits was used (Fig. 1). All perfusion equipment was
kept kitchen clean. Closed circuit perfusion was performed with 100 ml
of any of the perfusion media gassed throughout the experiment with
carbogen (5 % CO_2 + 95 % O_2). The perfusion media recirculated about
30 min in the apparatus in order to be equilibrated while preparation
of the isolated brain was performed. Arterial pressure was maintained
between 100 and 120 mm Hg as monitored continuously with a pressure
transducer (Statham P 23 Db). The perfusion rate was measured by means
of a burette. Bipolar electroencephalograms (EEG preamplifier Hellige
EE) were recorded from each hemisphere with two electrodes placed in
small depressions bilaterally in the bone of the parietal areas. The
perfusion experiments were continued only if the brains showed at the
most only a small decline in the spontaneous electrical activity and
the perfusion rate was higher than 2 ml/min throughout the first perfusion period of 30 min. Survival of the isolated brain was defined
as the time period during which the amplitude of the spontaneous EEG
was higher than 25 µV.

In order to achieve ischemic conditions the perfusion apparatus was
switched off for 1 min after a perfusion period of 30 min. A recovery
period of 2 min followed ischemia. The brains were plunged into liquid
nitrogen after the initial perfusion period of 30 min, after the ischemic period and after the recovery period, respectively.

Perfusion media. The fluorocarbon perfusion medium which contained
20 per cent (v/v) FC 43 and 4.8 per cent (w/v) of the nonionic surfactant Pluronic F 68 and 7 mM glucose in Krebs-Henseleit solution
(Dirks et al., 1980) was used in most experiments (Table 1).

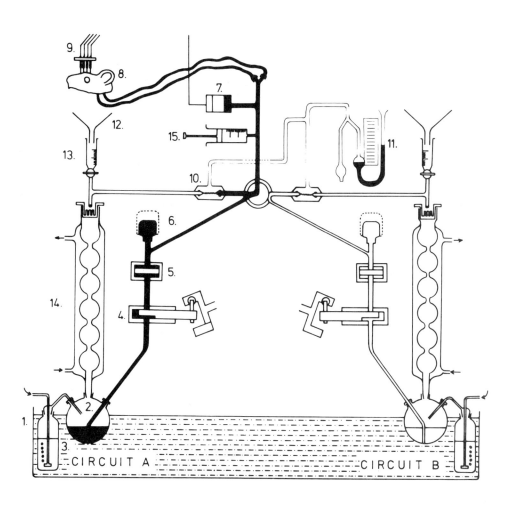

Fig. 1. Diagram of the perfusion apparatus with two circuits
         A and B.
         1. Water bath, 2. Reservoir, 3. Carbogen (95 % O$_2$
         and 5 % CO$_2$) humidified by bubbling through saline,
         4. Rotating piston pump, 5. Glass filter (pore
         width 40 - 90 μ), 6. Elastic reservoir to reduce
         pulse pressure, 7. Pressure transducer (Statham
         model P 23 Db), 8. Isolated rat brain, 9. Bipolar
         electrodes, 10. Starling resistor, 11. Manometer,
         12. Collecting funnel, 13. Calibrated tube for
         measuring perfusion rate, 14. Oxygenator, 15. Con-
         tinuous infusion apparatus.

TABLE 1   Composition and Properties of the Fluorocarbon Medium

Fluorocarbon FC 43[R]	$F_9C_4-N\langle{}^{C_4F_9}_{C_4F_9}$	20.0 ml
Pluronic F 68[R]	$HO(C_2H_4O)_x-(C_2H_3O)_y-(C_2H_4O)_xH$ CH_3	4.8 g
Glucose		140 mg
Krebs-Henseleit solution		to 100 ml
Oxygen content	(STPD, n = 5)	8.86 $\pm$ 0.43 ml/100 ml
Particle size distribution	0.1 μm	44 %
	0.1 - 0.4 μm	49.5 %
	0.4 μm	6.5 %
Viscosity	(range 2.95 - 3.24 cP)	3.13 cP
Osmolarity		310 mosmol

An artificial blood was used in a few experiments in order to compare the usefulness of the media. This medium consisted of well-washed bovine red cells, not older than 72 hours, suspended in Krebs-Henseleit solution containing 2 g per cent (w/v) bovine serum albumin and 7 mM glucose. The haematocrit of this preparation was 29.0 $\pm$ 1.6 per cent.

Determination of substrates in brain tissue.   Cerebral tissue was removed from the frozen brain at -20°C, weighed and extracted with HCl-methanol at that temperatur according to Folbergrova et al. (1972). The following substrates were measured enzymatically according to procedures given by Bergmeyer (1970): Creatine-phosphate, ATP, ADP, AMP, glycogen, glucose, pyruvate and lactate. Glucose-6-phosphate, fructose-6-phosphate and fructose-1,6-diphosphate were analyzed enzymatically by fluorometric methods reported by Lowry and Passonneau (1972). The values given in μmol/g wet weight of brain tissue were not corrected for the extracellular space.

Electronmicroscopic examination.   For electronmicroscopic examination brain tissue was fixed via the vascular system after a perfusion time of 3 hours using a formaldehyde-glutaraldehyde fixative according to Ito and Karnovsky (1968). Small tissue blocks were processed according to standard procedures. Sections stained with uranylacetate and lead citrate were examined with a Siemens Elmiskop I electron microscope.

RESULTS

Using this fluorocarbon emulsion for perfusion, the isolated rat brain
showed an EEG similar to that taken during perfusion with the artificial blood (Fig. 2). We found predominant beta activity and after a
quantitative EEG analysis a similar percentage of the frequency bands.

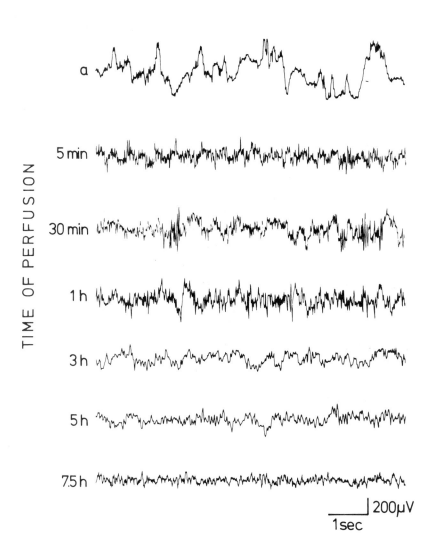

Fig. 2. Long survival time of the isolated rat brain per-
         fused with the fluorocarbon medium.
         a: EEG during preparation under surgical anesthesia.
         Interval samplings of the EEG are given during
         perfusion which lasted longer than 7 h 30 min.

An interruption of perfusion with the artificial blood for only 30 sec
caused almost a complete loss of the EEG. Brains perfused with the
artificial blood were not able to survive an ischemic period of 60 sec,
whereas in the case where perfusion with the fluorocarbon medium was
interrupted, EEG activity persisted for 60 sec (Fig. 3).

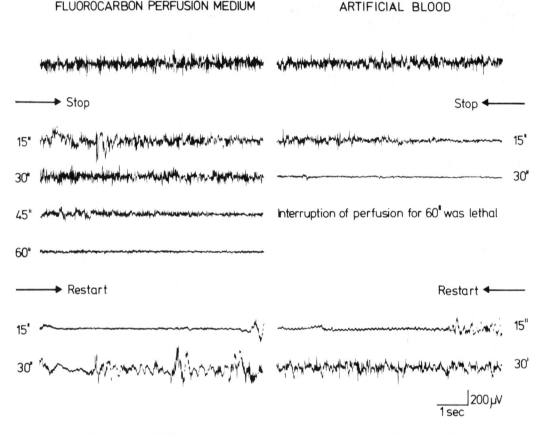

Fig. 3.   Effect of interruption of perfusion on the sponta-
           neous EEG after 30 min of perfusion.
           Between "Stop" and "Restart" the flow through the
           brain was interrupted (time is given in seconds).
           Notice the considerable time difference in the
           decline of the EEG when the fluorocarbon medium
           or the artificial blood were used.

Isolated brains perfused with the fluorocarbon medium for 3 hours were
examined by electron microscopy. The capillary bed appeared free from
mechanical obstructions such as fluorocarbon particles or blood clots.
No alteration of the capillary walls could be observed. The mitochondrial matrix and cristae were not disturbed and showed no signs of
swelling (Fig. 4).

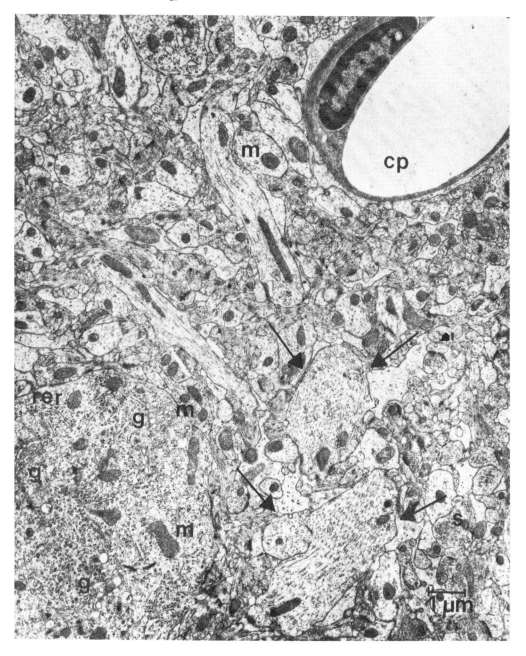

Fig. 4. Electron microscopic picture of the cortex of an
         isolated rat brain preparation perfused with flu-
         orocarbon medium for 3 hours. (cp) vascular endo-
         thelium, (arrows) cross sectioned axons, (s) synap-
         tic ending, (m) mitochondria, (g) Golgi complex,
         (rer) rough endoplasmic reticulum.

Using the isolated brain preparation for ischemic experiments, perfusion was stopped for 1 min after a perfusion period of 30 min.
A recovery period of 2 min followed ischemia. These perfusion experiments were carried out either without a drug or with methohexital
(0.2 mmol/l) added to the perfusion medium.

When the perfusion of the isolated brain was interrupted for 1 min,
the EEG disappeared irrespective of whether methohexital was added
to the perfusion medium or not, and it reappeared if the circulation
was restarted within 1 min. The EEG changes produced by the barbiturates, i.e. slow waves with high amplitudes, are typical for anesthesia. The adenylate energy charge (EC) determined after a perfusion
period of 30 min was comparable to those measured in intact rats
(Fig. 5).

The EC value is clearly reduced after 1 min of ischemia, but it is
less reduced when the barbiturate is present. After the recovery

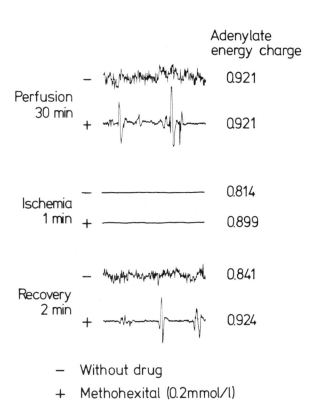

Fig. 5.   EEG and adenylate energy charge (EC) of the isolated rat brain.

period of 2 min the EC again reached the control level when methohexital was applied, but it was still lower than the control level
when no drug was added to the perfusion medium. After anesthesia with
methohexital we found no changes in the levels of the high-energy
phosphates (Fig. 6). Consequently, the EC was unaffected in anesthesia.

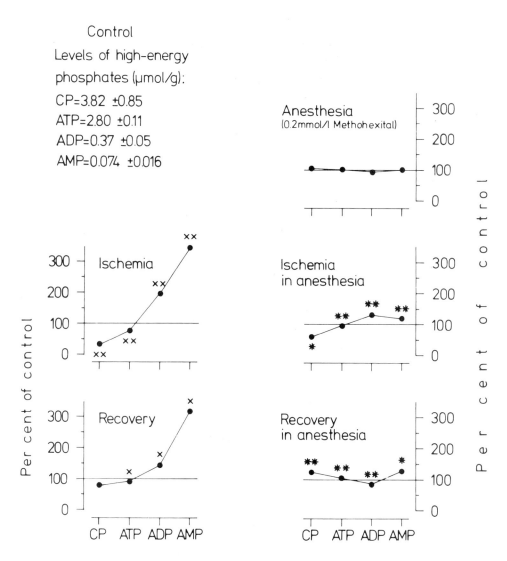

Fig. 6.   High energy phosphates in the isolated rat brain.
           After a perfusion period of 30 min (control) the
           flow to the brain was interrupted for 1 min (is-
           chemia), thereafter perfusion was continued for
           2 min (recovery). Means of 5 experiments ($\pm$ S.D.
           for control values). Different from control: $^{x}P<0.05$
           $^{xx}P<0.01$. Different from the corresponding value
           obtained without methohexital: $^{*}P<0.05$, $^{**}P<0.01$.

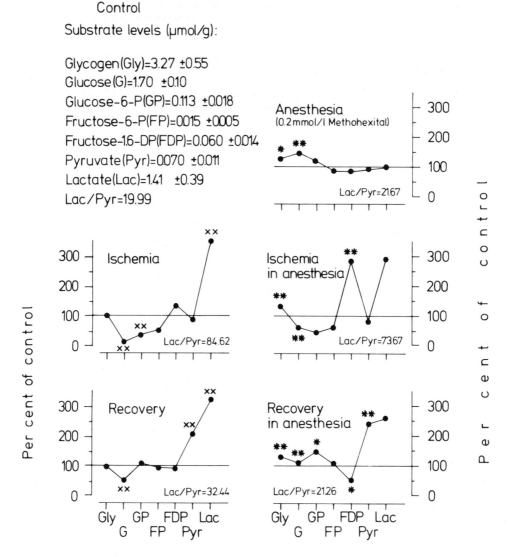

Control

Substrate levels (μmol/g):

Glycogen(Gly)=3.27 ±0.55
Glucose(G)=1.70 ±0.10
Glucose-6-P(GP)=0.113 ±0.018
Fructose-6-P(FP)=0.015 ±0.005
Fructose-1,6-DP(FDP)=0.060 ±0.014
Pyruvate(Pyr)=0.070 ±0.011
Lactate(Lac)=1.41 ±0.39
Lac/Pyr=19.99

Anesthesia
(0.2 mmol/l Methohexital)

Lac/Pyr=21.67

Ischemia

Lac/Pyr=84.62

Ischemia
in anesthesia

Lac/Pyr=73.67

Recovery

Lac/Pyr=32.44

Recovery
in anesthesia

Lac/Pyr=21.26

Fig. 7. Substrates of glycolysis in the isolated rat brain.
After a perfusion period of 30 min (control) the
flow to the brain was interrupted for 1 min (ischemia), thereafter perfusion was continued for
2 min (recovery). Means of 5 experiments ($\pm$ S.D.
for control values). Different from control:
$^{x}P < 0.05$, $^{xx}P < 0.01$. Different from the corresponding value obtained without methohexital: $^{*}P < 0.05$,
$^{**}P < 0.01$.

After the ischemic period without the anesthetic all organic phosphates given in Fig. 6 were significantly changed. The creatine-phosphate and ATP level were decreased, as well as ADP and AMP level increased. After the recovery period of 2 min the level of creatine-phosphate was no longer significantly diminished whereas the other phosphates were still clearly changed when compared to control conditions.

On the other hand, the high energy phosphate levels were significantly less altered after ischemia combined with anesthesia. The same was true after the recovery period using the anesthetic. The levels of creatine-phosphate and ATP were higher and the levels of ADP and AMP were lower than under recovery conditions without the anesthetic.

Some substrates of glycolysis were also measured (Fig. 7). The values obtained from isolated brains perfused for 30 min were used as controls. In anesthesia we found the glycogen and glucose level to be enhanced.

After ischemia without anesthesia glycogen is still unaffected. However, the glucose and glucose-6-phosphate level was significantly decreased and the lactate level is considerably increased under these conditions. Thus, the lactate/pyruvate ratio increased about four-fold.

After the recovery period the glucose level was still reduced. The pyruvate level also increased significantly and the lactate level remained high so that the lactate/pyruvate ratio decreased in comparison to ischemia.

The levels of glycolytic substrates measured after the ischemic period combined with anesthesia were clearly different from those measured in ischemia only. The glycogen level was elevated and the glucose level was less reduced in ischemia combined with anesthesia. Furthermore, the fructose-1,6-diphosphate level is significantly increased under these conditions clearly indicating that phosphofructokinase was activated.

After recovery of the brain in anesthesia the level of glycogen, glucose, glucose-6-phosphate and pyruvate were significantly higher than after recovery without the drug. The lactate/pyruvate ratio again reached the control level. The increase in glucose-6-phosphate and the decrease in fructose-1,6-diphosphate indicate an inhibition of phosphofructokinase activity under recovery conditions.

        DISCUSSION

The isolated perfused rat brain provides a method in which a total assessment of metabolic processes and electrical activity could be made by examining the brain. The EEG of the isolated rat brain may be used as a sensitive criterion of viability. Spontaneous EEG activity was detectable up to 10 hours (Krieglstein et al., 1972b). The recorded EEG revealed beta activity predominantly when no drug was applied. Drugs added to the perfusion medium produced specific (Rieger and Krieglstein, 1974; Krieglstein and Stock, 1975; Rieger et al., 1979) and dose-dependent EEG changes (Grüner et al., 1973; Bruns et al., 1978; Krieglstein et al., 1980). Furthermore, the energy state of the isolated rat brain was not different from that determined in rat and mouse brain in vivo (Table 2).

J. Krieglstein, B. Dirks and J. Hanke

<u>TABLE 2</u> High-Energy Phosphate Levels in the Isolated Rat
          Brain in Comparison to those Obtained from Rat
          and Mouse Brain in vivo

Brain preparation	Creatine-phosphate	ATP	ADP	AMP	$\frac{ATP}{ADP}$
Isolated perfused rat brain (a)	2.82 ± 0.12	2.37 ± 0.06	0.71 ± 0.02	0.19 ± 0.01	3.4
Rat brain in vivo (a)	2.57 ± 0.18	2.38 ± 0.05	0.78 ± 0.02	0.21 ± 0.01	3.1
Mouse brain in vivo (b)	2.43	2.36	0.91	0.21	2.6

Values (except ratios) are given in μmol/g wet tissue of whole brain,
means ± S.E.M. The isolated rat brain was perfused with the erythro-
cyte perfusion medium in this series.
(a) Krieglstein et al. (1972a), (b) Lowry et al. (1964).

In earlier experiments we used an artificial blood containing bovine
erythrocytes and bovine serum albumin for our perfusion experiments
(Krieglstein et al., 1972a). However, these physiological constituents
bring along with them substrates as for example lactate or various
enzyme activities. In order to overcome the disadvantages of the
erythrocytes in the perfusion medium, we developed a totally synthetic
perfusion medium with perfluorotributylamine (FC 43) as an oxygen
carrier. Because the fluorocarbon is not soluble in water an emulsion
has to be used. Emulsification was achieved by ultrasonic vibration.
Pluronic F 68 was used as a surfactant because it is atoxic, inert,
and, in addition, it behaves as an oncotic agent. The size of the
liquid particles in the emulsion is particularly important for its
stability. The average particle size of our medium is exactly within
the recommended range of 0.1 - 0.4 μm. Thus, the emulsion is stable
enough to be stored for several weeks in the refrigerator.

An ischemic period of 1 min obviously accelerates the glycolytic flux
rate and reduces the adenylate energy charge in the isolated perfused
rat brain as expected from experiments with rat brain in vivo (for a
review, see Siesjö, 1979). The barbiturate methohexital retards these
changes in energy reserves during ischemia. Similar results have been
reported by other authors (Lowry et al., 1964; Gatfield et al., 1966;
Brunner et al., 1971).

After the recovery period phosphofructokinase activity seems to be
clearly inhibited by methohexital. The results presented may suggest
that an inhibition of phosphofructokinase activity by the barbiturate
becomes clearly evident only when the enzyme is activated and substrate is sufficiently present.

The isolated perfused rat brain seems to be useful for studies on
energy metabolism and this under well defined conditions. In particular, a two-circuit apparatus (Fig. 1) offers the intriguing possibility of switching instantaneously from one perfusion medium to another,
for instance from a normoxic to an anoxic medium. Thus, this procedure

may also be suitable for experiments on hypoxia.

ACKNOWLEDGEMENTS

The experiments were carried out with the financial support of the
Deutsche Forschungsgemeinschaft and the Stiftung Volkswagenwerk.
The authors are indebted to Dr. N. Paul (Institut für Cytobiologie
und Cytopathologie, Marburg) for the electron microscopic analysis
of the brains and to Miss U. Hahn and Mrs. U. Lucas-Broermann for
valuable technical assistance.

REFERENCES

Andjus, R.K., K. Suhara, and H.A. Sloviter (1967). J. Appl. Physiol.,
22, 1033-1039.
Bergmeyer, H.U. (1970). Methoden der enzymatischen Analyse. Verlag
Chemie, Weinheim.
Brunner, E.A., J.V. Passonneau, and C. Molstadt (1971). J. Neurochem.,
18, 2301-2316.
Bruns, H., J. Krieglstein, and K. Wever (1978). Anaesthesist, 27,
557-561.
Dirks, B., J. Krieglstein, H.H. Lind, H. Rieger, and H. Schütz (1980).
J. Pharmac. Methods, in press.
Folbergrova, J., U. Ponten, and B.K. Siesjö (1974). J. Neurochem., 22,
1115-1125.
Gatfield, P.D., O.H. Lowry, D.W. Schulz, and J.V. Passonneau (1966).
J. Neurochem., 13, 185-195.
Grüner, J., J. Krieglstein, and H. Rieger (1973). Naunyn-Schmiedeberg's
Arch. Pharmacol., 277, 333-348.
Ito, S., and M.J. Karnovsky (1968). J. Cell. Biol., 39, 168a-169a.
Krieglstein, G., J. Krieglstein, and R. Stock (1972a). Naunyn-Schmiede-
berg's Arch. Pharmacol., 275, 124-134.
Krieglstein, G., J. Krieglstein, and W. Urban (1972b). J. Neurochem.,
19, 885-887.
Krieglstein, J., and R. Stock (1974). Psychopharmacologia (Berl.), 35,
169-177.
Krieglstein, J., and R. Stock (1975). Biochem. Pharmacol., 24, 1579-
1582.
Krieglstein, J., H. Rieger, and H. Schütz (1980). Biochem. Pharmacol.,
in press.
Lowry, O.H., and J.V. Passonneau (1972). A Flexible System of Enzymatic
Analysis. Academic Press, New York.
Lowry, O.H., J.V. Passonneau, F.X. Hasselberger, and D.W. Schulz
(1964). J. Biol. Chem., 239, 18-30.
Rieger, H., and J. Krieglstein (1974). Psychopharmacologia (Berl.),
39, 163-179.
Rieger, H., J. Krieglstein, and H. Schütz (1979). Pharmakopsychiat.,
12, 94-101.
Siesjö, B.K. (1978). Brain Energy Metabolism. John Wiley and Sons,
Chichester, New York, Brisbane, Toronto.
Woods, H.F., and M.B.H. Youdim (1977). Essays Neurochem. Neuropharma-
col., 2, 49-69.

DISCUSSION

Hudlicka: What is the oxygen carrying capacity of fluorocarbon medium which you were using?

Krieglstein: 8 ml/100 ml medium.

Hossmann: You used a very short period of ischemia in these experiments to demon-strate the changes between unanesthetized and barbiturate anesthetized animals. Dr. Siesjö, demonstrated after longer periods of ischemia going up to 30 min, that there is no difference whatsoever in the recovery between animals anesthetized and not anesthetized with barbiturates. I wonder if the changes which you see are actually due to the fact that barbiturates lower the metabolic rate to such an extent that after 1 min of ischemia brain metabolism is very little disturbed. If this is a fact, then it would be not very surprising that you have a faster recovery in the anesthetized animals.

Krieglstein: This is right. It was a little bit surprising for us to see that the influence of the ischemic effect is relatively small. You have to remember that the energy charge is not so much reduced, but it is significantly reduced.

Hossmann: Did you try longer periods of ischemia?

Krieglstein: No, we used this perfusion medium with fluorocarbon already a few months. In the beginning we used a simplified blood. The simplified blood did not allow longer ischemic periods. It is possible that longer ischemic periods are feasible by using other perfusion mediums.

Andjus: I have many questions, but I will make a selection. Most of my questions are of technical nature. We used hypothermia for the surgical procedure in our experiments. You use anesthesia. What was the reason for not using hypothermia? This was my first question. The second question goes to the temperature of the preparation. You were comparing in your study the results obtained from the iso-lated brain with the results of brain in vivo. For instance, the effect of ischemia and the recovery. I would like very much to know what is the temperature of the brain actually in the preparations, because this can cause a difference in results.

Krieglstein: You asked why we used anesthesia. We used your method before we used anesthesia and we saw that with your method the energy metabolism of the brain was very much influenced. It was very much different from the intact animal and rat brain in vivo.

Mandel: Perhaps, there are some other questions?

Krieglstein: The question concerning the temperature of the isolated brain seems important.

Mandel: I see. All the technical points are very important.

Andjus: I do not think it's a technical question. The temperature is below 30°. So you are comparing a brain at a temperature below 30° with a brain at 38° and the question of effects of 30 seconds of ischemia or some minutes is different. You can not compare it because the metabolic rate is lower below 30°. And you expect differences concerning the time.

Krieglstein: Dr. Andjus, there are several problems involved. Not only pharmaco-logical and biochemical problems, but also ethical problems. If the brain temperature is 37°, one can ask: has the brain pain? What about pain for this preparation. And therefore we remained with the temperature below 30°.

Mandel: I think we are a bit behind our schedule. I have one single question: I am a bit aware about the evaluation of the energy content. Because from our experience, the energy compound which drops extremely fast, much faster than ATP, is phosphocreatine. Did you measure phosphocreatine?

Krieglstein: Yes.

Animal Models in Experimental Gerontopsychiatry

S. Hoyer, L. Frölich and M. Hof

Institut für Pathochemie und Allgemeine Neurochemie im Zentrum
Pathologie der Universität Heidelberg, Heidelberg,
Federal Republic of Germany

ABSTRACT

Two main but different brain diseases are responsible for gerontopsychiatric disorders in men: multi infarct and degenerative processes. The latter are characterized by neurofibrillary tangles. Vincristine is able to produce neurofibrillary
tangles. It also inhibits RNA synthesis in the brain. Investigations were performed
to study the effect of vincristine upon the glycolytic and oxidative breakdown of
glucose and the energy metabolism in the brain which mostly is involved in degenerative brain processes and which is closely related to protein metabolism. It could
be found that vincristine inhibits the glycolytic flux by means of inhibiting the
flux-controlling enzyme phosphofructokinase. These results are in agreement with
findings in patients suffering from Alzheimer's disease in whom a very low phosphofructokinase activity was found. The vincristine model seems to be useful in experimental gerontopsychiatry.

KEYWORDS

Gerontopsychiatric disorders; brain energy metabolism; phosphofructokinase;
vincristine.

INTRODUCTION

Animal models in experimental medicine should fulfil the condition that they are
closely related to human diseases. In gerontopsychiatry, the main disease is dementia, mostly due to primary degenerative brain processes and far less frequently
caused by cerebrovascular disturbances (Tomlinson, Blessed and Roth, 1970; Jellinger, 1976) Table 1).

35

TABLE 1   Classification of the dementias on the basis of morphological findings in brain tissue.

About 90 % of the dementias can be classified morphologically, of these show:

60 % degenerative

20 - 25 % vascular (multi infarct)

15 - 20 % both, degenerative and vascular damages in brain tissue

These different types of dementias are associated with different variations in blood flow and metabolism of the brain. It could be shown that in the initial phase of the dementias the metabolic rate of glucose was primarily disturbed, while blood flow and oxygen consumption of the brain were within normal ranges (Fig. 1).

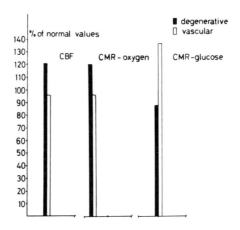

CBF, CMR-oxygen and CMR-glucose expressed as percentages of normal values in dementia due to degenerative and vascular (multi infarct) brain diseases at the beginning of the dementia process

In primary degenerative dementia a deficit in brain glucose could be found and in multi infarct dementia a surplus of glucose was measured (Hoyer, 1978 a). The imbalance between oxygen and glucose became obvious in both dementia types and was in the latter similar to cerebral hypoxia (Kogure and coworkers, 1970; Hamer and coworkers 1976 and 1978). It could be furthermore demonstrated that in patients suffering from dementias not classified into primary degenerative or multi infarct types, and irrespective of the time course of the disease, cerebral blood flow was predominantly decreased in only 17.5 %, while prevalent decreases in the metabolic rates of oxygen and/or glucose were present in 68 % (Hoyer, 1970).
These results along with the morphological changes mentioned above let it thus seem unlikely that the primary pathophysiological damage in dementia would be due to cerebral circulation. There is more support for the assumption that the relevant

and most frequent types of dementia would be more due to disturbance in brain tissue itself, i. e. in various biological systems in the brain cells responsible for
brain metabolism and controlling it. In dementia research, it thus would not be
appropriate to perform animal experimental investigations by influencing the
transportation system, i. e. cerebral circulation and/or the composition of the
blood perfusing the brain, as this would be necessary and useful in terms of other
aspects of experimental brain research.

EXPERIMENTAL

The measurements of cerebral blood flow, CMR-oxygen and CMR-glucose reported here,
were performed of the Kety-Schmidt technique (1948) as modified by Bernsmeier and
Siemons (1953). Patients suffering from dementia due to brain infarcts, brain
tumors, head injuries, cerebral infections, exogenous or endogenous intoxications,
were excluded from the investigations or not reported here. The measurements were
carried out in untreated patients under steady state conditions of mean arterial
blood pressure and in normoxia and normocapnia.
The investigations concerning the metabolites in brain cortex were performed as
randomized studies. The animals were intubated or tracheotomized and artificially
ventilated with 0.5 vol % halothane and a mixture of nitrous oxide/oxygen 70 : 30 %.
Under steady state conditions of normal mean arterial blood pressure, normoxia,
normocapnia and normothermia, the brains of the animals were frozen in situ via a
scalp funnel by means of liquid nitrogen. All animals were excluded in which it
was not possible to maintain the steady state conditions. The biochemical analysis
of the compounds of the glycolytic chain, the citric acid cycle and the energy
pool were carried out according to Lowry and Passonneau (1972) and Folbergrova,
MacMillan and Siesjö (1972 a and 1972 b).

RESULTS AND DISCUSSION

On the basis of the inhomogeneous variations in brain blood flow and metabolism
in dementia patients, some animal models will be discussed which may throw light
on the underlying neurobiochemical disturbances in dementia.
As a hypothesis, one may assume that the decreased cerebral metabolic rate of glucose as measured in patients suffering from primary degenerative dementia is due
to either a disturbance in the mechanism for glucose transport across the blood-
brain barrier or due to a disturbance in the breakdown of glucose in the glycolytic chain and/or the citric acid cycle.
The transport of glucose from the arterial blood across the blood-brain barrier
into the brain is carrier-mediated. This carrier can be partially inhibited by
phlorizin and more strongly by phloretin (Oldendorf, 1971; Pardridge and Oldendorf, 1975 and 1977). The intraperitoneal or intravenous application of 20 mmol/l
/kg body weight phlorizin, resulted in a statistically significant increase of the
concentration of glucose-6-phosphate and in statistically significant decreases of
both, fructose-1, 6-diphosphate and lactate, as compared to a control group in
brain cortex of cats (Fig. 2).
These results indicate that phlorizin also seems to decrease the breakdown of glucose in the glycolytic chain. The activity of the flux-controlling enzyme phosphofructokinase is obviously inhibited. It might seem more likely that the increased
concentration of glucose-6-phosphate is not due to an increased hexokinase activity but also due to the decreased phosphofructokinase activity (Newsholme and
Start, 1973). Although the glycolytic flux runs at a lower level as compared to
normal conditions, the concentrations of the compounds of both, the citric acid
cycle and the energy pool, were not changed. This may indicate that substrates
other than glucose may be metabolized in the brain to yield energy.

S. Hoyer, L. Frölich and M. Hof

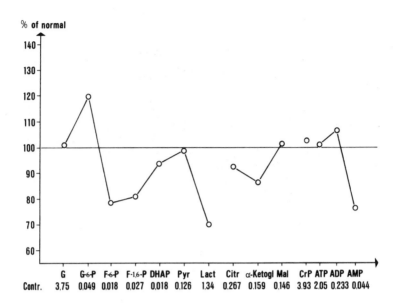

CORTICAL GRAY MATTER CONCENTRATIONS OF THE INTERMEDIATES OF THE GLYCOLYTIC CHAIN,
THE CITRIC ACID CYCLE AND THE ENERGY POOL AFTER THE APPLICATION OF PHLORIZIN IN CATS

THE 100% - NIVEAU CORRESPONDS TO THE CONTROL GROUP

Preliminary results of measurements of blood flow, oxygen consumption, glucose uptake and lactate release of the brain in dogs, showed that phlorizin decreased
both the metabolic rates of glucose and lactate, whereas the oxygen consumption
remained unchanged as compared to controls. These metabolic changes corresponded
not only with the findings in the cortical gray matter but were also similar to
those in dementia patients mentioned above. In the latter,either a cerebral com-
bustion of amino acids from the arterial blood or of endogenous brain substrates,
instead of the lacking glucose, could be found (Hoyer, 1975).
In other dementia patients, a normal cerebral metabolic rate of glucose along with
a markedly increased lactate/glucose index could be observed. It may be speculated
that an impairment of the oxidative glucose metabolism which takes place in the
mitochondria may be responsible for an increased lactacidosis in the cell and thus
for the increased lactate output from the brain. As a model, isonicotinic acid
hydrazide (INH) which influences transamination, oxidative deamination and
decarboxylation of amino acids by means of the inhibition of vitamin B_6 in the
citric acid cycle (Meister, 1965),could imitate these variations in animal experiments.
Findings of brain blood flow and metabolism in another group of dementia patients
were characterized by a predominant decrease in cerebral oxygen consumption at
normal oxygen concentration in arterial blood. The decrease in the cerebral metabolic rate of oxygen might not only be explained by the accompanying decrease in
cerebral blood flow which fell to a much lesser extent than CMR-oxygen. As a reason for these variations,damage to the respiratory chain may be postulated. In
experimental animals,the function of the respiratory chain can be impaired by
means of cyanide which inhibits the cytochrome oxidase reaction. In animals,
the intraperitoneal injection of 200 mg/kg body weight INH as well as the subcutaneous application of 7 mg/kg body weight cyanide,produce also a diminution
of both amplitude and frequency in the EEG, as does phlorizin (10 to 20 mmol/l/kg
body weight (Hoyer, 1978 b) (Fig. 3).

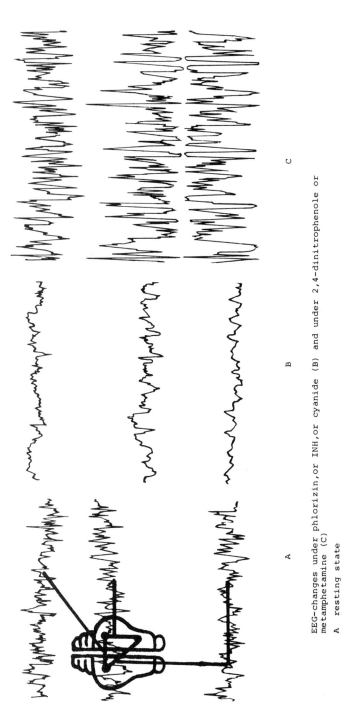

EEG-changes under phlorizin,or INH,or cyanide (B) and under 2,4-dinitrophenole or metamphetamine (C)

A resting state

In dementia patients showing clinically productive symptoms such as a delirium, or a Korsakow syndrome or a hallucinosis, cerebral blood flow and the metabolic rates of oxygen and glucose were found to be pathologically elevated if no or only a slight brain atrophy was present. One may assume that the augmentations in brain blood flow and metabolism are due to a pathological activation in the metabolism of neurotransmitters in the brain or due to an uncoupling of oxidative phosphorylation. Cerebral blood flow and the cerebral metabolic rate of oxygen increased markedly after amphetamine application and in immobilization stress, as could be demonstrated by Carlsson, Hägerdal and Siesjö (1975 a and 1975 b).

The EEG changes after the application of either metamphetamine (9 mg/kg body weight i. p.) or 2,4-dinitrophenol (20 mg/kg body weight i. p.) were similar. Both substances produce an activation of amplitude and frequency which is reversible 90 to 120 minutes after the application (Fig. 3). In brain cortex of cats, the intraperitoneal application of 2,4-dinitrophenol (20 mg/kg body weight) produced a statistically significant decrease in the concentration of glucose-6-phosphate and statistically significant increases of both, fructose-1, 6-phosphate and lactate, indicating an increase in the activity of the flux-controlling enzyme phosphofructokinase (Fig. 4).

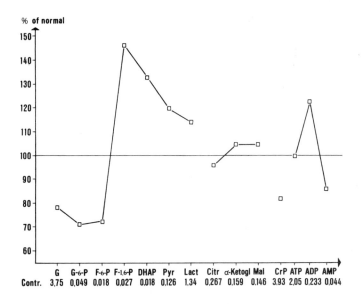

CORTICAL GRAY MATTER CONCENTRATIONS OF THE INTERMEDIATES OF THE GLYCOLYTIC CHAIN, THE CITRIC ACID CYCLE AND THE ENERGY POOL AFTER THE APPLICATION OF 2,4 - DINITRO-PHENOLE IN CATS

THE 100% - NIVEAU CORRESPONDS TO THE CONTROL GROUP

According to Carlsson, Hägerdal and Siesjö (1976) it seems not to be likely that the increase in body temperature of 1.2 °C on average, after the application of 2,4-dinitrophenol, may influence the concentrations of the glycolytic metabolites, since the arterial blood pressure, paO_2 and pa CO_2 were in steady state and did not change as compared to controls.

Although these animal models yielded information on cerebral metabolic variations after damage to important biological systems in the brain, and although they seem to be closely related to variations in dementia patients, there can be no doubt that these models suffer from some disadvantages. There are namely two more important points which should be regarded in gerontopsychiatric research in experimental animals. Firstly, dementia in patients is generally not an acute,but a subchronic or chronic brain disease. Secondly, the dominating type of dementia in patients is morphologically associated with neurofibrillary tangles. But animals do not habitually develop such neurofibrillary tangles in their ageing process. It therefore would be necessary to produce artificially such morphological variations in experimental animals. Beside aluminium (Crapper and Dalton, 1973) vincristine, the alkaloid from Vinca rosea can produce neurofibrillary tangles in humans as well as in experimental animals (Schochet and coworkers, 1968; Seil and Lampert, 1968; Wisniewski, Terry and Hirano, 1970). Biochemical studies showed an inhibition of RNA synthesis by vincristine in mouse brain (Agustin and Creasey, 1967). Protein biosynthesis is a process consuming large amounts of energy. The brain derives its energy mainly from the oxidation of glucose. A disturbance in neuronal biosynthesis could therefore lead one to suspect also a disturbance in the glucose and energy metabolism of the brain.

We performed acute and subchronic experiments with vincristine in rats. Acute animals were treated over two days, the first day with 0.2 mg/kg body weight, the second day with 0.1 mg/kg body weight intraperitoneally. Subchronic animals received 0.1 mg/kg body weight per day intraperitoneally over a period of 21 days.

After a two-day application of vincristine the animals did not show any behavioral or neurological symptoms as compared to controls. In brain cortex,the concentration of fructose-1,6-diphosphate was decreased to a statistically significant extent. There were some more but smaller variations in the glycolytic chain intermediates but without any statistical significance (Fig. 5).

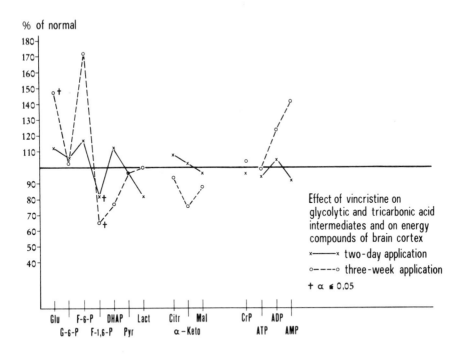

Effect of vincristine on glycolytic and tricarbonic acid intermediates and on energy compounds of brain cortex

x———x two-day application

o————o three-week application

+ α ≤ 0.05

After a three-week application of vincristine a more severe disturbance in the glycolytic breakdown of glucose in brain cortex could be found. The concentration of glucose was markedly increased and the concentration of fructose-1,6-diphosphate was significantly decreased. The qualitative changes in the intermediates of the glycolytic chain were similar,but much more extensive after a three-week application than after a two-day application (Fig. 5). Thus, it seems to be obvious that vincristine inhibits the flux-controlling enzyme phosphofructokinase. The increase of glucose along with the normal concentration of glucose-6-phosphate indicates also an inhibition of the hexokinase step. These results in experimental animals seem to be in agreement with findings in patients suffering from Alzheimer's disease in whom a very low phosphofructokinase activity was found (Bowen, Spillane, Curzon and coworkers, 1979). It may be assumed that a decrease in the glycolytic flux would lead to an impoverishment of glucoplastic amino acids such as glutamate, alanine etc., which derive from glucose and which are formed in the citric acid cycle whose activity would seem also to be decreased in the subchronic experiments. Since these amino acids are also building blocks for protein synthesis one could assume that the biosynthesis of proteins in the brain, which are necessary and responsible for biological information, is decreased.

It was remarkable that there was no energy deficit as measured by creatine phosphate, ATP, ADP, and AMP although the decreased flux of glucose through the glycolytic chain should produce an energy deficit in the brain. Since the activity of the citric acid cycle seems to be decreased,too,it seems to be unlikely that amino acids could be combusted in the brain to yield energy. The present results do not show why the energy pool remains unchanged. If the consumption of the energy-rich compounds could be assumed to be decreased unter these experimental conditions, then there would be one more reason for the decreased biosynthesis of proteins in the brain.

Ultrastructural studies[1] in parietal cortical gray matter, hypothalamus, cervical ganglion (C 5) and spinal motor ganglion cells (C 5 - C 7) revealed a moderate degranulation and disruption of the rough endoplasmatic reticulum and an increase of polysomes after a three-week application of vincristine. These findings indicate a damage in protein metabolism which corresponds to a certain degree to the metabolic changes mentioned above.

The morphological and biochemical changes in the brain of the subchronic animals were associated with behavioral and neurological reactions. The responsiveness of the animals to exogenous stimuli appeared to be markedly diminished. The animals appeared to be dulled. They showed ataxia and in a lesser extent paresis of the hind legs.

Experimental gerontopsychiatry is just in the beginning of its development. At present, there is more speculation than hard facts, in contrast to other fields in experimental brain research. Nevertheless, there are some promising models which may lead to a better understanding of the pathobiochemical variations in the brains of dementia patients.

This may be of great importance since there is no doubt that life expectancy is increasing in the population of the civilized countries. An old desire of mankind is hereby fulfilled. But if human longevity would mean a life with reduced mental faculties (i. e. dementia), then the meaningfulness of this desire is questionable.

[1] Dr. Benedikt Volk, Dept. of Neuropathology, University of Heidelberg, performed the ultrastructural studies in a total of 5 animals (3 subchronic application of vincristine, 2 controls). The animals were perfused by means of a solution of 3 % glutaraldehyde 0.14 molar in Sorensen phosphate buffer pH 7.3. For these investigations and for the permittance to demonstrate the results we are indebted to Dr. Volk.

REFERENCES

Agustin, B. M., and W. A. Creasy (1967). Vinca alkaloids and the synthesis of RNA in mouse brain. Nature, 215, 965 - 966.

Bernsmeier, A., and K. Siemons (1953). Die Messung der Hirndurchblutung mit der Stickoxydul-Methode. Pflüger's Arch. ges. Physiol., 258, 149 - 162.

Bowen, D. M., J. A. Spillane, G. Curzon, W. Meier-Ruge, P. White, M. J. Goodhart, P. Iwangoff, and A. N. Davison (1979/I). Accelerated ageing or selective neuronal loss as an important cause of dementia. Lancet, 11 - 14.

Carlsson, C., M. Hägerdal, and B. K. Siesjö (1975 a). Influence of amphetamine sulphate on cerebral blood flow and metabolism. Acta physiol. scand., 94, 128 - 129.

Carlsson, C., M. Hägerdal, and B. K. Sisejö (1975 b). Increase in cerebral oxygen uptake and blood flow in immobilization stress. Acta physiol. scand., 95, 206 - 208.

Carlsson, S., M. Hägerdal, and B. K. Siesjö (1976). The effect of hyperthermia upon oxygen consumption and upon organic phosphates, glycolytic metabolites, citric acid cycle intermediates and associated amino acids in rat cerebral cortex. J. Neurochem., 26, 1001 - 1006.

Crapper, D. R., and A. J. Dalton (1973). Aluminum induced neurofibrillary degeneration, brain electrical activity and alterations in acquisition and retention. Physiol. Behav., 10, 935 - 945.

Folbergrova, J., V. MacMillan, and B. K. Siesjö (1972 a). The effect of moderate and marked hypercapnia upon the energy state and upon the cytoplasmatic NADH/ NAD$^+$ ratio of the rat brain. J. Neurochem., 19, 2497 - 2505.

Folbergrova, J., V. MacMillan, and B. K. Siesjö (1972 b). The effect of hypercapnic acidosis upon some glycolytic and Krebs cycle - associated intermediates in the rat brain. J. Neurochem., 19, 2505 - 2517.

Hamer, J., S. Hoyer, E. Alberti, and F. Weinhardt (1976). Cerebral blood flow and oxidative brain metabolism during and after moderate and profound arterial hypoxaemia. Acta neurochir., 33, 141 - 150.

Hamer, J., K. Wiedemann, H. Berlet, F. Weinhardt, and S. Hoyer (1978). Cerebral glucose and energy metabolism, cerebral oxygen consumption and blood flow in arterial hypoxaemia. Acta neurochir., 44, 151 - 160.

Hoyer, S. (1970). Der Hirnstoffwechsel und die Häufigkeit cerebraler Durchblutungsstörungen beim organischen Psychosyndrom. Dtsch. Z. Nervenheilk., 197, 285 - 292.

Hoyer, S. (1975). Cerebral blood flow and oxidative metabolism in dementia patients. Symp. on Behavior and the Aging Brain. Durham, N. C.

Hoyer, S. (1978 a). Blood flow and oxidative metabolism of the brain in different phases of dementia. In: R. Katzman, R. D. Terry, Katherine L. Bick (Eds.): Alzheimer's disease: Senile dementia and related disorders (Aging Vol. 7). New York; Raven Press pp. 219 - 226.

Hoyer, S. (1978 b). Überlegungen zum Führen eines Wirkungsnachweises von Pharmaka beim organischen Psychosyndrom. Arzneim.-Forsch./Drug Res. 28 (II), 2312 - 2315.

Jellinger, K. (1976). Neuropathological aspects of dementias resulting from abnormal blood and cerebrospinal fluid dynamics. Acta Neurol. Belg., 76, 83 - 102.

Kety, S. S., and C. F. Schmidt (1948). The nitrous oxide method for the quantitative determination of cerebral blood flow in man: theory, procedure and normal values. J. clin. Invest.,27, 467 - 483.

Kogure, K., P. Scheinberg, O. M. Reinmuth, M. Fujishima, and R. Busto (1970). Mechanisms of cerebral vasodilatation in hypoxia. J. appl. Physiol., 29, 223 - 229.

Lowry, O. H., and J. Passonneau (1972). A flexible system of enzymatic analysis. New York; Academic Press.

Meister, A. (1965). Biochemistry of the amino acids. Vol. 1, 2nd ed. New York, London; Academic Press pp. 375 - 413.

Newsholme, E. A., and C. Start (1973). Regulation in metabolism. London; Wiley.

Oldendorf, W. H. (1971). Brain uptake of radiolabeled amino acids, amines, and hexoses after arterial injection. Am. J. Physiol., 221, 1629 - 1639.

Pardridge, W. M., and W. H. Oldendorf (1975). Kinetics of blood-brain barrier transport of hexoses. Biochim. Biophys. Acta, 382, 377 - 392.

Pardridge, W. M., and W. H. Oldendorf (1977). Transport of metabolic substrates through the blood-brain barrier. J. Neurochem., 28, 5 - 12.

Schochet, S. S. jr., P. W. Lampert, and K. M. Earle (1968). Neuronal changes induced by intrathecal vincristine sulfate. J. Neuropath. exp. Neurol., 27, 645 - 658.

Seil, F. J., and P. W. Lampert (1968). Neurofibrillary tangles induced by vincristine and vinblastine sulfate in central and peripheral neurons in vitro. Exp. Neurol., 21, 219 - 230.

Tomlinson, B. E., G. Blessed, and M. Roth (1970). Observations on the brains of demented old people. J. Neurol. Sci., 11, 205 - 242.

Wisniewski, H., R. D. Terry, and A. Hirano (1970). Neurofibrillary pathology. J. Neuropath. exp. Neurol., 29, 163 - 176.

DISCUSSION

Mandel: Although we are a bit behind our schedule, it is not so bad because fortunately or unfortunately, Dr. Siesjö is not here. So that we can have our coffee break for 15 minutes.

Thank you Dr. Hoyer for your very interesting presentation. Questions or comments?

Vogel: I have a question: You showed very large differences of biochemical parameters in brain due to vincristine. Is this confined only to brain or are other organs like liver, kidneys and so on, influenced in a similar manner?

Hoyer: Well, we did not investigate other organs. Our interest is directed towards the brain. But it can be assumed that other organs are influenced, too. Since, if you applicate this vincristine intraperitoneally or subcutaneously, you many observe general and severe disturbances in the animals (which we discarded from this study), and therefore we changed our methods. Now we applicate this vincristine over a burr hole in the extradural space at very low amounts and as a very low volume. The first investigations showed the same results as shown here.

Mandel: May I ask you a question? You suggested a hypothesis that mitochondrial metabolism may be altered. Have you some direct evidence about this?

Hoyer: I think it is no question that the glycolytic metabolism is the metabolism of the cytoplasm and the oxydative metabolism is the metabolism of the mitochondria, and we know some substances which may influence the oxydative metabolism and from this we conclude that it's the damage of the mitochondrial function.

Experimental Occlusion of the Middle Cerebral Artery in Cats

K.-A. Hossmann

Max-Planck-Institut für Hirnforschung, Forschungsstelle für
Hirnkreislaufforschung, Ostmerheimstr. 200,
5000 Köln-Merheim (91), Federal Republic of Germany

ABSTRACT

In cats, the middle cerebral artery was occluded for 1 to 4 hours using a transorbital approach. EEG, brain volume, cortical impedance, brain water, electrolyte content and substrates of the energy-producing metabolism were measured and correlated with regional cerebral blood flow. A threshold of 10 - 15 ml/100 g/min was established for the development of ischemic brain edema. Ischemia was progressive when blood flow decreased below this level (critical ischemia), but it was reversible when flow remained above the threshold (non-critical ischemia). A therapeutic amelioration of experimental stroke was attempted by raising perfusion pressure, reducing vascular resistance, decreasing blood viscosity, and by metabolic inhibition with barbiturates or hypothermia. None of these approaches was successful. The results are interpreted in regard to the pathophysiology of experimental stroke, and further strategies for the investigation of therapy are proposed.

KEYWORDS

Middle cerebral artery occlusion; experimental stroke; cats; blood flow; thresholds of ischemia; therapy.

INTRODUCTION

In the statistics of mortality and morbidity, cerebro-vascular disease and stroke rank among the three most frequent clinical disorders (Zülch, 1971). The great interest in the therapeutic amelioration of this disease has prompted numerous attempts for the development of experimental models in which therapeutic procedures can be tested under standardized, reproducible conditions. Unfortunately, very few of these models mimic the actual clinical situation. The survival time of healthy, pre-treated animals under hypoxic conditions, the energy state following decapitation or the metabolic rate of the normoxic brain under pharmacological influence are parameters which have little or nothing to do with the pathophysiology of cerebro-vascular disorders. Of greater relevance are those experimental situations, in which the blood supply to the brain is critically reduced. Among the various experimental models, two groups can be distinguished which differ in regard to the technical difficulty of the experimental procedure and the reliability of the ischemic impact. On one hand are those procedures in which a major supplying artery such as

47

the carotid artery is occluded <u>extracranially</u>, and on the other hand are experimental models in which a cerebral artery is ligated <u>intracranially</u>. It is obvious,
that the extracranial ligation of the carotid artery is a simple operation, but in
most animal species this does not result in critical cerebral ischemia because the
circulus Willisi in healthy animals ensures full compensation by collateral blood
supply from the contralateral side. Only in the gerbil, in which the circulus
Willisi is incomplete, ligation of the carotid artery results in unilateral ischemia in about 30 to 40 % of the experiments (Levine and Payan, 1966). In rats occlusion of the cerebral artery causes unilateral brain damage when an additional
anoxic stress supervenes, e.g. in the Levine model in which unilateral carotid occlusion is combined with several transient anoxic episodes until neurological
symptoms appear (Levine, 1960). Another, more recent approach is the carotid ligation in spontaneously hypertensive rats (Fujishima and co-workers, 1977). These
animals exhibit diffuse vascular changes which, from a pathophysiological point of
view, resemble advanced atherosclerosis and which prevent an adequate collateral
blood supply to the contralateral hemisphere after unilateral carotid occlusion.

Although the extracranial carotid-occlusion models are technically easy to accom-
plish, they have the disadvantage that the resulting ischemic impact varies considerably from animal to animal, and that - for this reason - large series of experiments have to be performed in order to test pharmacological or other therapeutic procedures. A more reliable ischemic impact can be obtained by <u>intracranial</u>
occlusion of a cerebral artery. In general, the middle cerebral artery is used for
this purpose because in most species it supplies the larger portion of the hemisphere. Several techniques have been developed for this purpose: Embolization of
the middle cerebral artery with steel balls (Penry and Netsky, 1960), blood clots
(Hill and co-workers, 1955) or plastic material (Molinari, 1970; Bremer and co-
workers, 1975) via the carotid artery; temporal craniotomy with subsequent exposure
of the middle cerebral artery using a lateral approach (Anthony and co-workers,
1963); and the transorbital approach according to the technique of Hudgins and
Garcia (1970). From a technical point of view, embolism of the middle cerebral
artery is relatively easy, but it has the disadvantage that the location of the
embolus may vary, and the size of the infarct, accordingly. The temporal approach
is also a relatively simple operation but in order to expose the middle cerebral
artery, the temporal lobe has to be dislocated which may produce traumatic lesions
and brain edema, complicating the ischemic impact. The transorbital approach is
technically by far the most difficult procedure. An eye ball has to be removed, and
microneurosurgical techniques using an operating microscope are necessary for the
application of a vessel clip to the middle cerebral artery in the depth of the
orbit via the foramen opticum. The advantage, on the other hand, is that by careful procedure, the brain is not traumatized and that the middle cerebral artery can
be occluded permanently or transiently at precisely the same segment under visual
control. This is the reason that more and more laboratories are using this technique for the study of the pathophysiology and, more recently, also of the therapy
of experimental stroke (Hayakawa and Waltz, 1975; Michenfelder and co-workers,
1976; Symon and co-workers, 1975b). The only disadvantage is the fact that because
of the great technical difficulty it is not possible to investigate large series
of animals for pharmacological screening purposes. For this reason most authors
perform the experiments in such a way that a maximum of information is drawn from
a minimum number of animals, i.e. by using multidisciplinary techniques for the
investigation of the resulting ischemic impact.

In the following, our experience with this model will be discussed. During the
past years, more than 150 animals have been investigated in our laboratory for the
study of the pathophysiology, biochemistry and therapy of experimental stroke.
Most of the data obtained have been published or submitted for publication elsewhere (Blöink and co-workers, 1979; Hossmann and Schuier, 1979a, 1979b, 1980;
Schuier and Hossmann, 1980). In the following a summary of these investigations is
given.

RESULTS

Surgical Procedures

Experiments were carried out in adult cats. The animals were anesthetized either
with a single intraperitoneal injection of pentobarbital (Nembutal, 30 mg/kg) or
with 70 % nitrous oxide and 0.5 % halothane. The animals were immobilized and artificially ventilated throughout the experiment. Body temperature was kept constant at 37° C, arterial PCO_2 close to 30 mm Hg and arterial PO_2 above 100 mm Hg.
The animals were placed in a stereotaxic frame, the left eye ball was removed and
the foramen opticum was enlarged using a dental drill. Under the operating microscope the dura was split, the middle cerebral artery exposed at its origin from
the carotid artery and freed from the arachnoid membrane with fine needles. Occlusion of the vessel was performed using a Mayfield clip proximal to the origin of
the ascending branches to the basal ganglia. Blood flow was measured using the
intracardiac microsphere injection technique (Rudolph and Heymann, 1967). This
technique was chosen because it allowed the correlation of blood flow and tissue
constituents in the same tissue sample. A catheter was placed into the left ventricle of the heart via the brachial or femoral artery, and 15 ± 3 μ microspheres
labeled with different nuclides were injected before ischemia, 15 minutes after
the occlusion of the middle cerebral artery, and at the end of the experiments. A
reference blood sample was withdrawn at a calibrated speed from the femoral artery.
The animals were kept alive for 1 to 4 hours, and EEG, brain volume, and cortical
impedance were continuously monitored. At the end of the experiments Evans blue or
carbon black was injected for tracing the extent of ischemia, the brain was removed, and dissected in a moist chamber. Samples were taken from ischemic and non-
ischemic areas and processed for blood flow, brain water and brain electrolytes.
In one series of experiments the brain was frozen in situ, dissected under irri-
gation with liquid nitrogen and processed for brain tissue osmolality and for biochemical substrates in addition to the above mentioned procedures.

Cerebral Blood Flow

Although the middle cerebral artery was occluded under visual control, the decrease
in blood flow in the territory of this vessel varied considerably from animal to
animal. 15 minutes after vascular occlusion, cortical blood flow ranged between 4
and 50 ml/100 g/min (mean 21.3 $\pm$ 5.6), and white matter flow between 6 and 31 ml/
100 g/min (mean 19.3 $\pm$ 3.8). Despite the great variability of the individual flow
values, in none of the animals complete cessation of blood flow was observed. This
is of great pathophysiological importance because, in contrast to cardiac arrest or
to experimental models of complete ischemia, middle cerebral artery occlusion apparently does not lead to a full stop of blood flow. In consequence, a continuous
though reduced exchange of substrates and fluid between brain and blood is present,
which presumably is responsible for the rapid beginning of brain swelling and the
relatively good preservation of energy metabolism, as described below.

Flow changes were also observed in the borderzone of the middle cerebral artery
territory, and the more distant parts of the ipsilateral hemisphere. In these regions blood flow initially also decreased, but subsequently generally improved. In
the opposite hemisphere changes in blood flow were minor, indicating that during
the initial 4 hours of ischemia a diaschitic disturbance of contralateral hemo-
dynamics did not occur.

The great scatter of flow values in the territory of the middle cerebral artery
demonstrates, that even in healthy animals under reproducible experimental conditions, considerable differences in the collateralization of the occluded vessel
exist. Without precise knowledge of the individual flow rates, therefore, an inter-

pretation of the physiological, biochemical and morphological consequences of
middle cerebral artery occlusion is not possible. In the following, such a correlation is attempted.

Size of Infarcts

The size of the ischemic territory following middle cerebral artery occlusion was
determined by the "single dye passage"-technique (Weber and co-workers, 1974), i.e.
the absence of staining following intra-arterial injection of a bolus of carbon
black or Evans blue. When blood flow in the center of the occluded middle cerebral
artery territory was plotted against the size of the infarct, a distinct relationship was noted. In all animals, in which ischemia covered more than 50 % of the
MCA territory, blood flow was below 18 ml/100 g/min. This value is very close to
the critical threshold for maintenance of ion homeostasis, as will be described
below, and indicates that collateral blood supply is not able to maintain blood
flow above this critical level when more than half of the MCA territory is ischemic.

Electroencephalogram

EEG within a few seconds after middle cerebral artery occlusion decreased considerably in amplitude over the affected hemisphere. Calculation of EEG intensity by
Fourier transform revealed a decrease to about 20 % of the control which corresponds to an amplitude reduction of more than 50 %. EEG frequency content, on the
other hand, was little affected. The relative intensity of the fast frequency
bands was very close to the pre-ischemic value, indicating that the EEG flattened
but did not slow down. When EEG intensity was correlated with blood flow, a linear
relationship over the whole range of flow values was observed. This is in contrast
to the suppression of evoked potentials which is definitely threshold-dependent
(Branston and co-workers, 1974). EEG activity, in consequence, decreased in parallel with blood flow, indicating that with increasing density of ischemia an increasing portion of the excitable neuropil was inhibited.

EEG of the contralateral hemisphere was little affected. During the four hours'
observation period, neither EEG amplitude nor EEG frequency significantly changed.
Electrocortical diaschisis, in consequence, was not a prominent feature during the
initial phase of infarct development.

Water and Electrolyte Content

In contrast to the EEG, a definite threshold was observed for disturbances of
water and electrolyte homeostasis. At flow values above 10 - 15 ml/100 g/min, no
significant changes in water or electrolyte content of brain tissue were observed,
although disturbances of EEG activity were present. At flow rates below this level,
however, severe ischemic brain edema developed. Within 4 hours water content of
the cortex in the territory of the middle cerebral artery increased from 80.7 ± 0.4
to 83.0 ± 0.3 % wet weight. Water increase was accompanied by a parallel increase
of sodium from 262 ± 9 to 454 ± 13 and a decrease of potassium from 442 ± 20 to
305 ± 32 meq/kg dry weight. The opposite shifts of the cations were reflected by
changes of the Na/K ratio which dramatically increased from 0.6 ± 0.03 to 1.55 ±
0.17.

Ischemic brain edema started almost immediately after vascular occlusion. This
could be demonstrated by continuous monitoring of brain volume with an induction
transducer, which revealed a beginning of brain swelling within less than 1 minute

after the onset of ischemia. The electrolyte shifts in the cerebral cortex were accompanied by a shift of fluid from the extra- into the intracellular compartment, as demonstrated by recording cortical impedance which is a function of the size of the extracellular space. Using the Maxwell equation which describes the relationship between impedance and cell volume, the changes in the size of the extracellular space could be calculated. According to this equation extracellular space within 5 minutes shrank from 19.8 to 14.6 %, followed by a more slowly narrowing to 11.4 % within 2 hours. Cell hydrops, in consequence, developed more rapidly and more dramatically than could be concluded from the changes in net water uptake. This may explain the considerable swelling, particularly of glial cell processes, which have been observed by electronmicroscopy before (Little and co-workers, 1976).

Water inhibition during ischemic brain swelling was mainly due to an increase in tissue osmolality. Using a method described by Arieff and co-workers (1972), an increase in tissue osmolality by 16 - 22 mosmol/kg wet weight was observed in the territory of the MCA. This value corresponds numerically to the increase in lactate (see below) and suggests that the accumulation of this product in the ischemic territory is of importance for the development of brain edema. However, other osmotically active particles such as electrolytes, glucose and phosphate also change during ischemia. This may be the reason for the fact that despite the relationship between lactate and tissue osmolality, a significant correlation between lactate content and increase in water was not observed.

The swelling of glial cell processes associated with the development of brain edema caused a gradual compression of microcirculation . This can be concluded from the fact that in the presence of brain swelling ischemia was progressive (critical ischemia). In animals in which edema was absent, i.e. in which blood flow remained above the critical threshold for disturbances of ion homeostasis, blood flow - in contrast - gradually improved, presumably as a consequence of improved collateralization of the ischemic territory (non-critical ischemia). It is obvious, that tissue necrosis can not be prevented when blood flow gradually deteriorates. This leads to the conclusion, that brain edema is a critical phenomenon in the development of stroke, and that prevention of infarcts requires the prevention of this complication.

Energy Metabolism

Within 4 hours of ischemia, creatine phosphate in the territory of the occluded middle cerebral artery decreased from 2.96 ± 0.32 to 1.44 ± 0.11 μmol/g wet weight. ATP, during the same period, decreased from 2.00 ± 0.19 to 1.10 ± 0.09 μmol/g wet weight. This decrease is surprisingly small when compared to the dramatic changes in water and electrolyte balance and when compared to complete ischemia, in which energy-producing metabolism breaks completely down within a few minutes (Ljunggren and co-workers, 1974). On the other hand, in animals with non-critical ischemia, in which brain edema was absent, the concentration of high energy phosphates was only slightly higher than in animals with critical ischemia. Involvement of energy metabolism, in consequence, is not a critical phenomenon for the development of ischemic brain edema.

The relatively well preserved energy state of the brain in regions in which blood flow was far below the critical threshold for maintenance of tissue integrity is difficult to explain. One factor may be a shutdown of cortical activity, leading to a saving of the energy demands of the tissue (Bito and Myers, 1972). As has been described above, EEG amplitude decreases at substantially higher flow values than those causing a breakdown of energy metabolism, and it is reasonable to assume that with decreased cortical activity the energy requirements of the brain also decrease. The high concentrations of energy-rich phosphates, in consequence, would

then reflect a decrease in energy consumption rather than maintenance of energy
production. This may also explain the fact that in experiments performed by
Ginsberg and co-workers (1977), glucose consumption in the territory of the middle
cerebral artery almost ceased.

From a pathophysiological point of view the hypothesis of spontaneous inhibition
of energy requirements under conditions of critical ischemia is of great practical
interest. If the ischemic brain shuts off its energy requirements, therapeutic in-
tervention by a metabolic inhibition would be unnecessary or even harmful. As will
be described below, this actually seems to be the case.

Therapeutic Interventions

The only causal therapy of ischemia is the restoration of blood flow. In the presence of a permanently occluded vessel, recirculation of the ischemic territory is
possible only by collateral blood supply, mainly by the pial anastomotic arteries.
A critical factor for the efficacy of collateral blood supply is vascular resistance. As has been described above, a decrease of blood flow below a critical
threshold of 10 to 15 ml/100 g/min initiates ischemic brain edema which, in turn,
leads to a progressing compression of microcirculation and thus an increase in vascular resistance. This presumably is the reason for the fact that edema and not
the breakdown of the energy metabolism or functional suppression is the critical
factor for permanent irreversible tissue damage. Therapy, in consequence, should
be directed towards an increase of blood flow above the critical threshold for the
induction of edema because only in the presence of a low vascular resistance collateral blood supply can be expected to gradually improve.

From a theoretical point of view, there are several possibilities to achieve this
goal. Blood flow may be improved by increasing perfusion pressure, by decreasing
vascular resistance or by decreasing the viscosity of the circulating blood. In
addition, a lowering of the threshold for the initiation of edema, e.g. by metabolic inhibition, might prevent this critical complication at low flow values. According to this theoretical concept, we have tested various therapeutic procedures in
a large series of animals. The therapeutic effect was evaluated by estimating ischemic brain edema and by comparing blood flow 2 hours after the onset of ischemia
with the flow rate immediately after vascular occlusion. Every animal, in consequence, served as its own control.

The results obtained so far are depressingly negative. Neither a decrease of vascular tone by sympathectomy or prostacyclin, a decrease of blood viscosity by defibrinogenation, or hemodilution, or metabolic inhibition by barbiturate or hypothermia caused a significant improvement of blood flow or an amelioration of ischemic brain edema. Even hemodilution with 10 % dextran which distinctly raised blood
flow was not able to prevent brain edema. The reason for this discrepancy is presumably the fact, that by hemodilution oxygen content of the blood decreases and
therefore oxygen availability does not improve. A deterioration of brain edema was
also observed following treatment by barbiturate or hypothermia, presumably because
of a decrease in blood pressure which fell far below the values observed in non-
treated animals. This finding is in contrast to previous observations of a beneficial effect of barbiturates on the size and occurrence of infarcts following middle
cerebral artery occlusion in primates (Hoff and co-workers, 1975). It is unlikely
that there are species differences between primates and cats, and it is therefore
suggested that the beneficial effect of barbiturates observed before was due to the
prevention of complicating side effects, rather than of the primary ischemic impact. Such side effects could be provoked by the development of vasogenic brain
edema which after 4 to 6 hours of ischemia supervenes and which, in addition to
the primary ischemic brain edema, may cause a further deterioration of blood flow

in the borderzone of the infarct or even critical intracranial hypertension (Ng and Nimmannitya, 1970).

Negative results were also obtained by improving perfusion pressure. Increase of the arterial blood pressure by about 50 mm Hg caused a distinct increase in blood flow in the non-ischemic contralateral hemisphere, but not in the ischemic territory itself. This finding is surprising because autoregulation in the center of the ischemic territory is lost (Sundt and co-workers, 1976; Symon and co-workers, 1975a), and an increase in perfusion pressure should increase blood flow in this region. A possible explanation may be that the blood pressure rise caused an autoregulatory constriction of the (non-ischemic) pial arteries which are responsible for the collateral blood supply to the ischemic territory. This might shut off rather than improve the collateral blood flow to the territory of the occluded vessel.

CONCLUSIONS

The present data and results from various other laboratories using the same experimental model have demonstrated that stroke following experimental vascular occlusion is a threshold phenomenon which presumably is related to the development of ischemic brain edema rather than to a breakdown of the energy-producing metabolism (Branston and co-workers, 1974; Heiss and co-workers, 1976; Held and co-workers, 1975; Little and co-workers, 1976; Morawetz and co-workers, 1978; Symon and co-workers, 1979). Prevention of edema, therefore, seems to be the prerequisite for a successful treatment of this condition. The complexity of the interrelationship between ischemia, edema and regional disturbances of flow regulation makes it almost impossible to design a therapeutic approach based on observations in healthy animals or in animals under non-ischemic conditions. This stresses the importance of using experimental models for the design of therapeutic procedures which precisely mimic the acutal clinical situation. Transorbital middle cerebral artery occlusion is a very useful model for this purpose and the results obtained indicate that, in fact, many of the generally applied therapeutic procedures are inefficient or may even deteriorate the normal pathophysiological sequel. However, the experimental model being now firmly established, it should be possible by systematic exploration, to identify those drugs or procedures which have a possibly beneficial effect. The greatest chance for a successful amelioration of ischemic infarcts is given to those approaches which cause a prevention of the early development of ischemic brain edema. It therefore seems to be of utmost importance to first clarify the pathophysiology of this dangerous complication in order to design further therapeutic strategies.

ACKNOWLEDGEMENT

The careful editing of this manuscript by Mrs. Langer is gratefully acknowledged.

REFERENCES

Anthony, L.U., S. Goldring, J.L. O'Leary and H.G. Schwartz (1963). Experimental cerebrovascular occlusion in dog. Arch.Neurol., 8, 515-527.
Arieff, A.I., C.R. Kleeman, A. Keushkerian and H. Bagdoyan (1972). Brain tissue osmolality: Method of determination and variations in hyper- and hypo-osmolar states. J.Lab.Clin.Med., 79, 334-343.
Bito, L.Z. and R.E. Myers (1972). On the physiological response of the cerebral cortex to acute stress (reversible asphyxia). J.Physiol. (Lond), 221, 349-370.

Blöink, M., V. Hossmann and K.-A. Hossmann (1979). Treatment of experimental infarcts following middle cerebral artery occlusion in cats. In A. Bès and G.
Géraud,(Ed.), Circulation cérébrale, Toulouse, pp. 85-87.

Branston, N.M, L. Symon, H.A. Crockard and E. Pasztor (1974). Relationship between
the cortical evoked potential and local cortical blood flow following acute
middle cerebral artery occlusion in the baboon. Exp.Neurol., 45, 195-208.

Bremer, A.M., O. Watanabe and R.S. Bourke (1975). Artificial embolization of the
middle cerebral artery in the primates. Stroke, 6, 387-390.

Fujishima, M., Y. Nakatomi, K. Tamaki, J. Ogata and T. Omae (1977). Cerebral isch-
emia induced by bilateral carotid occlusion in spontaneously hypertensive rats.
Supratentorial and infratentorial metabolism and arterial acid-base-balance. J.
Neurol.Sci., 33, 1-11.

Ginsberg, M.D., M. Reivich and A. Giandomenico (1977). Altered local brain glucose
utilization during focal ischemia: hypometabolism, hypermetabolism, and
diaschisis. Stroke, 8, 131-131.

Hayakawa, T. and A.G. Waltz (1975). Immediate effects of cerebral ischemia: Evo-
lution and resolution of neurological deficits after experimental occlusion of
one middle cerebral artery in conscious cats. Stroke, 6, 321-327.

Heiss, W.-D., T. Hayakawa, and A.G. Waltz (1976). Cortical neuronal function during
ischemia. Effects of occlusion of one middle cerebral artery on single-unit
activity in cats. Arch.Neurol., 33, 813-820.

Held, K., O. Jacobsen, K. Kraft and W. Berghoff (1975). Regional cerebral metabo-
lism in experimental brain infarction. In T.W. Langfitt, L.C. McHenry, Jr., M.
Reivich and H. Wollman (Ed.), Cerebral Circulation and Metabolism, Springer
Verlag, New York, Heidelberg, Berlin. pp. 82-84.

Hill, N.C., C.H. Millikan, K.G. Wakim and G.P. Sayre (1955). Studies in cerebrovascular disease; experimental production of cerebral infarction by intracarotid
injection of homologous blood clot; preliminary report. Proc.Staff Meet. Mayo
Clin., 30, 625-633.

Hoff, J.T., A.L. Smith, H.L. Hankinson and S.L. Nielsen (1975). Barbiturate protection from cerebral infarction in primates. Stroke, 6, 28-33.

Hossmann, K.-A. and F.J. Schuier (1979a). Metabolic (cytotoxic) type of brain edema
following middle cerebral artery occlusion in cats. In T.R. Price and E. Nelson
(Ed.), Cerebrovascular Diseases, Raven Press, New York. pp. 141-165.

Hossmann, K.-A. and F.J. Schuier (1979b). Pathophysiology of stroke edema. In K.J.
Zülch, W. Kaufmann, K.-A. Hossmann and V. Hossmann (Ed.), Brain and Heart Infarct II. Springer Verlag, Berlin-Heidelberg-New York, pp. 119-129.

Hossmann, K.-A. and F.J. Schuier (1980). Experimental brain infarcts in cats. I.
Pathophysiological observations. Stroke, submitted for publication.

Hudgins, W.R. and J.H. Garcia (1970). Transorbital approach to the middle cerebral
artery of the squirrel monkey: A technique for experimental cerebral infarction
applicable to ultrastructural studies. Stroke, 1, 107-111.

Levine, S. (1960). Anoxic-ischemic encephalopathy in rats. Am.J.Pathol, 36, 1-17.

Levine, S. and H. Payan (1966). Effects of ischemia and other procedures on the
brain and retina of the gerbil (meriones unguiculatus). Exp.Neurol., 16, 255-262.

Little, J.R., F.W.L. Kerr and T.M. Sundt, Jr. (1976). Microcirculatory obstruction
in focal cerebral ischemia: An electron microscopic investigation in monkeys.
Stroke, 7, 25-30.

Ljunggren, B., H. Schutz and B.K. Siesjö (1974). Changes in the energy state and
acid-base parameters of the rat brain during complete compression ischemia.
Brain Res., 73, 277-289.

Michenfelder, J.D., J.H. Milde and T.M. Sundt, Jr. (1976). Cerebral protection by
barbiturate anesthesia. Use after middle cerebral artery occlusion in Java
monkeys. Arch.Neurol., 33, 345-350.

Molinari, G.F. (1970). Experimental cerebral infarction. I. Selective segmental
occlusion of intracranial arteries in the dog. Stroke, 1, 224-231.

Morawetz, R.B., U. DeGirolami, R.G. Ojemann, F.W. Marcoux and R.M. Crowell (1978).
Cerebral blood flow determined by hydrogen clearance during middle cerebral

artery occlusion in unanesthetized monkeys. Stroke, 9, 143-149.

Ng, L.K.Y. and J. Nimmannitya (1970). Massive cerebral infarction with severe brain swelling: A clinicopathological study. Stroke, 1, 158-163.

Penry, J.K. and M.G. Netsky (1960). Experimental embolic occlusion of a single leptomeningeal artery. Arch.Neurol., 3, 391-398.

Rudolph, A.M. and M.A. Heymann (1967). The circulation of the fetus in utero: Methods for studying distribution of blood flow, cardiac output and organ blood flow. Circ.Res., 21, 163-184.

Schuier, F.J. and K.-A. Hossmann (1980). Experimental brain infarcts in cats. II. Ischemic brain edema. Stroke, submitted for publication.

Sundt, T.M., Jr., R.E. Anderson and F.W. Sharbrough (1976). Effect of hypocapnia, hypercapnia, and blood pressure on NADH fluorescence, electrical activity, and blood flow in normal and partially ischemic monkey cortex. J.Neurochem., 27, 1125-1153.

Symon, L., N.M. Branston and O. Chikovani (1979). Ischemic brain edema following middle cerebral artery occlusion in baboons. Relationship between regional cerebral water content and blood flow at 1 to 2 hours. Stroke, 10, 184-191.

Symon, L., H.A. Crockard, N.W.C. Dorsch, N.M. Branston and H. Juhasz (1975a). Local cerebral blood flow and vascular reactivity in a chronic stable stroke in baboons. Stroke, 6, 482-492.

Symon, L., N.W.C. Dorsch and H.A. Crockard (1975b). The production and clinical features of a chronic stroke model in experimental primates. Stroke, 6, 476-481.

Weber, R., M. Furuse, M. Brock and H. Dietz (1974). The single dye passage. A new technique for the study of cerebral blood flow distribution. Stroke, 5, 247-251.

Zülch, K.J. (1971). Hemorrhage, thrombosis, embolism. In J. Minckler (Ed.), Pathology of the Nervous System, Vol. 2, McGraw-Hill Book Comp., New York. pp.1499-1536.

DISCUSSION

Mandel: Thank you Dr. Hossmann for your stimulating presentation. This paper is open for discussion.

Nitz: Did you see in your experiments the so-called steal-phenomenon using typical vasodilators like papaverine?

Hossmann: We have not yet used the vasodilators in our model, but we know from other laboratories that such phenomena have been observed.

Berlet: You have pointed out the difficulties in delineating the area of the infarct.

Hossmann: We have expressed the volume of the infarct after middle cerebral artery occlusion in percent of the volume of the hemisphere. It is in the range between 18 and 62 % of the hemisphere volume.

Müller: Do you have any experience with corticosteroids or with high concentration of glucose or with diuretics?

Hossmann: We have some experience with osmotherapy where we have used Manitol to increase the osmolarity of the circulating blood, but we could not prevent edema. We do not have experience with corticosteroids but there are numerous experiments of other groups which were not successful either. The reason in my opinion is the following: corticosteroids seem to act particularly on the vasogenic type of edema and not so much on the cytotoxic type. Following middle cerebral artery occlusion, edema initially is of the cytotoxic type. Only after an interval of 6 - 12 hours, vasogenic type of edema supervenes. At this stage, the ischemic tissue is already necrotic. Corticosteroids therefore may prevent secondary changes due to vasogenic edema, but will not prevent the development of an infarct.

Müller: Which kind of hemodilution did you use?

Hossmann: This was isovolemic hemodilution with 10 % Rheomacrodex dextrane.

Seiffge: In your experiments you have very bad pharmacological conditions for blood flow. Your attempts to reduce blood viscosity only goes to reduce red cell aggregation by hemodilution or defibrinogenation but only on one slide you have shown as well an increase in lactate. An increase in lactate or decrease in pH will give you very rigid red cells. Have you ever tried to reduce this?

Hossmann: Well, we have not tried, but I think that's a very reasonable suggestion because the rigidity of the red cells certainly contributes to the increase in viscosity. This is one of the approaches which should be tested in the future.

Rudolphi: To which extent did the blood gases change during your hemodilution?

Hossmann: Blood gases do not change but the oxygen content changes; it falls in parallel with the decrease of hematocrit down to 15 %.

Mandel: Could you in a chronic experiment arrive to a situation that the edema decreases?

Hossmann: We have not performed such experiments, but there is a paper by O'Brien and Waltz who demonstrated, in fact, a gradual increase of water content and then a gradual decline. This was probably due to the development and resolution of the vasogenic type of edema which is a delayed type of edema. It's our impression that vasogenic edema only develops under the conditions of tissue necrosis, i.e. when we have already an infarct. The swelling which we can see after a few days is an indicator of a secondary complication subsequent to the primary infarct. By treating or by influencing the edema, you may influence the secondary complications, but it will not be possible to influence the primary infarct.

Mandel: But actually in human pathology, we have a feeling that we are always dealing with the primary phenomenon of edema which produces additional alterations and then during the recovery, we think that the recovery is partially due to the disappearance of this edema. In the models we should have something parallel to what occurs in human pathology.

Hossmann: You are perfectly right, that the recovery is related to the resolution of vasogenic type of edema, but this will not reverse the infarct. It is the impact of the vasogenic type of edema on healthy brain tissue which is not infarcted, e.g. by relief of intracranial pressure.

Ostrowski: May I come back to one of your first slides? You showed us an ink slide. What can you say about the distribution of this dye-stuff. Is it in the blood vessels or also in the neurons?

Hossmann: No, it is in the blood vessels. It's the technique which has been described by Brock and it is called the "single dye passage". A bolus of carbon black is injected into the heart (into the left ventricle) and the animal is killed after 15 seconds, that means after a single passage of the dye.

Ostrowski: May I then join question to Prof. Sokoloff? Are you sure that you are measuring glucose utilization or are you only measuring blood flow with your radioactivity in brain?

Sokoloff: We are measuring glucose utilization. This is true for several reasons: One reason is that because we use a pulse and then wait a long time, we eliminate any influence of blood flow. We have direct proof of that. If we use another analogue of glucose, 3-O-methylglucose which is distributed by the blood just the same as deoxyglucose and is transported across the blood-brain barrier by the same carrier which transports glucose and deoxyglucose, but does not get phosphorylated, you don't see anything like what you see with deoxyglucose. The only difference is that one is phosphorylated. If we measure blood flow, methylglucose would give the same picture.

GENERAL DISCUSSION

Mandel: To profit from this general discussion, it will be useful to reconsider the problems, because it is obvious that you will leave this session and it will be most fruitful if you can leave the session with at least two or three new good ideas: So we should reconsider what we have dealt with and what we would like to learn. Two questions can be raised: What is hypoxia and what is aging? There is a possibility to discuss the problems as how far we are convinced that the main aging problem is the problem of hypoxia or what is the part of hypoxia and what is the part of aging of the tissue with all kinds of cellular alterations which are the consequence of aging.

A second point that we would like to have are suitable models to answer the questions what is hypoxia, what is aging and what are the means of therapy. We have proposad several models and each model has its limitations and its advantages. I think that it will be very fruitful to work out for each model which was proposed, what is the advantage and what is the limitation. The third point is the problem of methodology in our investigations. In this respect, we have several excellent proposals, for instance the proposal to use deoxyglucose. This leads us to consider what is the relative importance of different parameters what we have to investigate: which are blood flow, energy metabolism, cellular alterations and substrate availability. I think that if we could get an answer on each of these problems, we will learn something very important. Finally the problem can not be what will be the best therapy because up to now I think "therapie nulla est" but what in the opinion of people who are here would be the best way to look for therapy.

So, if you like, we can open the discussion.

Hoyer: I would like to open the discussion with the question: What is the definition of hypoxia? I think, we can't talk about this without any definition, and there are many different definitions. Perhaps Dr. Sokoloff and Dr. Hossmann will give us an answer to this.

Hossmann: From the pathophysiological point of view hypoxia is a mismatch between the oxygen needs of the tissue and the oxygen supply. That means whenever the oxygen needs of the tissue are higher than the oxygen supply, hypoxia ensues. This can be ascertained either by oxygen histograms by oxygen sensitive microelectrodes or by determination of the glucose/oxygen uptake ratio because under conditions of decreased oxygen supply anaerobic glycolysis is stimulated and this leads to an unproportionally high increase of glucose uptake.

Sokoloff: I would make the definition perhaps a little bit more specific in chemical terms. Most of the processes going on in tissues are parts of a chain of reactions. There are reaction sequences, and under normal circumstances, a certain reaction in a sequence is the rate limiting step that sets the rate for the whole pathway. Anytime, a substance becomes limiting in concentration, so that another step becomes rate-limiting, then you have a deficiency. So I would say that any time the oxygen level gets so low that its reduction becomes rate-limiting, you have hypoxia.

Mandel: Yes, I would say that my feeling is that actually what we are interested in is obviously oxygen supply; it is obviously the disturbances and sequences of different reactions, but the main problem, so far as we are interested in animals, is the supply of energy and the supply of substrate to produce certain amino acids. It seems to be that we are judging the degree of hypoxia according to the degree of energy supply or a supply of substrate from glucose metabolism necessary to produce amino acids.

Worcel: I would like to summarize from a naive point of view: my conclusion from
the session is that there are two problems: a circulatory problem and a metabolic
problem. I will put it in single terms: stroke and dementia. What concerns the
circulatory problem, the stroke problem, the consequence of the reduction of
oxygen supply is a metabolic effect that you measure either by internal deoxyglucose or by any other end product. But my question is: in any pathological or
experimental situation, when we just think in terms of stroke: what is the limiting step that you would interested in modifying in order to avoid metabolic
consequences for the brain. My conclusion is that it is some step in circulation.
I do not know where it is. Is it in the arteries, is it in the microcirculation,
but I feel that the limiting step is there and there we have to act.

Mandel: Other comments concerning hypoxia?

Sokoloff: I might amplify on what I said and give an example. What happens in
the cells is that the substrates are oxidized and the $NAD^{(+)}$ is reduced. There is
a whole sequence of steps in the electron transport chain going all way to the
reduction of oxygen. The speed of reaction, the oxidation by oxygen is very fast
and occurs with a very low level of oxygen that is not rate limiting normally.
The rate limiting step is probably the reoxidation of the reduced $NAD^{(+)}$. Now, if
you lower the oxygen, you slow up the cytochrome oxidase reaction, but you do not
change anything at first, because the step is so fast anyway that you slow it up
without changing the rate limiting step. Now, eventually, if you lower the oxygen
enough, what will becoming limiting is the cytochrome oxidase step, and the whole
chain will become reduced and you have an accumulation of reduced $NAD^{(+)}$. That
will change the redox state of the whole cell. That will have implications, not
only to ATP formation, but who knows what other reactions which are going on in
the cells are going to be affected by changing redox potentials. So, there is a
specific example of what I mean by hypoxia; you have changed the whole metabolic
balance of the cells, and the effect may have a variety of consequences which
follow reduction of the electron transport chain.
When $NAD^{(+)}$ is in too reduced state, there are many other reactions which are
affected other than ATP generation. Substances which are normally in an oxidized
state are now getting reduced. So that's a very complicated process.

Mandel: That's an excellent point, but I should say that extremely important the
production of $NAD^{(+)}$ is. We are producing a lot of NADH by drinking alcohol and
by giving barbiturates, but there is still a cell capacity to overcome this increase
of NADH and this, I think, is a fundamental point which we can reach now. This
means we have to think also, when we are looking for the aging problem which was
considered in parallel to hypoxia, that we should take under consideration that
hypoxia occurs in older people, in older brains, where we can already expect that
there are some or many cellular alterations. I would like to mention some of our
former studies on a tissue like lens for which we can not say that it can be
hypoxic, because there is no circulation. It's however one of the best models of
aging. It's a cellular model where we can see exactly the same alterations which
were reported here as aging alterations of the brain. That is alteration of glucose
metabolism, of enzyme biosynthesis, of the pool of amino acids, of RNA synthesis.

Now, if somebody would like to comment on hypoxia and aging, or we can go to the
second point, which concerns different models, because going home we will start to
work again and we will ponder the question: which model do we accept for further
investigations. Are there some comments or questions concerning the animal models?

Rudolphi: I would like to ask the experts on ischemia whether they have a model
for the study of micromultiple infarction?

Hoyer: I think it is necessary to differentiate between these two large groups:
the primary degenerative group and the multiinfarct dementia group. I think we
have some good models or good ideas on models for the primary degenerative group.
But I wonder if we have similar good ideas for models on the multiinfarct group.
I think that radiation may perform similar changes. Haymaker did some investigations years before and he found that the vessels react with a swelling in the
arterioles and the capillaries and I think he found small infarcts spreading over
the whole brain, but if this is similar in any way to multiinfarct, I do not know.

Mandel: Other questions or comments?

Martorana: I have a question to Dr. Hossmann. What would you expect a compound
to do in your model, to prove efficacy?

Hossmann: Well, to express it in a very naive way: to open the collaterals. This
is our major problem. In the brain the collateral supply to the middle cerebral
artery is by Henbuers arteries which are pial anastomoses on the surface of the
cortex, and the blood supply through these vessels has to be increased. The
problem is the following: these arteries originate at a point where the brain is
not ischemic, and therefore, they are under normal cerebrovascular control.
Moreover we need a reaction which is different from that of the healthy brain. They
should dilate although the vessels in the surrounding not ischemic territory
should constrict, because otherwise one would produce steal effects. I wonder if
this could be done just by superfusion of the cortical surface with vasoactive
agents or by sympathectomy because we know that the sympathetic tone of these
arteries is higher than in the intracellular vessels.

Martorana: Isn't sympathectomy too drastic. Would it be possible to use
phenoxybenzamine or an alpha blocker?

Hossmann: Yes, this has been done but the results as far as I know are not very
encouraging.

Sokoloff: Are we sure that these collaterals are not already maximally dilated
and that we are limited simply by the anatomical size and by the number of big
vessels.

Hossmann: I am not convinced that from an anatomical point of view, the vessels
should vary so much. I would expect that the number of collateral vessels is more
or less the same in all animals. But they are not maximally dilated, because in
the region from where they originate, there is no ischemia and no acidosis.
Acidosis is in the center of the infarct, and there the vessels, of course, are
dilated. But from where they originate, there is no acidosis and they should have
a normal tone.

Sokoloff: But hasn't it been evident that there is an excessive blood flow
surrounding the infarcted area?

Hossmann: Yes, you are right. There is an increase of blood flow but in the
center of the infarct. Cytotoxic edema develops which causes such an increase in

vascular resistance that even in the presence of a better blood supply flow
decreases.

Hudlicka: Did you try to test the effect of hypercapnia which is known to produce
vasodilation particularly in the small arterioles or in the small arteries?

Hossmann: We did not test this but there are many publications about this particular
question. For some time hyperventilation has been advocated to get something what
has been called "reverse steal phenomenon", this means increased perfusion in the
dilated vessels of the ischemic territory and decreased perfusion in the healthy
vessels which constrict during hyperventilation. But then serious reports came up
which just showed the opposite effect and therefore these experiments have not
been conducted.

Mandel: I would like to ask a question concerning this topic. Is there any model
of progressive occlusion of vessels which can reproduce what is happening actually
in vivo when during a progressive occlusion the collaterial circulation develops?

Hossmann: I think you are perfectly right, that during a more gradual occlusion,
the situation may be different. Our animal model is a model of acute occlusion
after metabolism. That's the clinical counterpart. However, I strongly feel that
pathophysiological principles like flow thresholds, are valid also for a gradual
occlusion.

Mandel: Extreme situation . . .

Hossmann: Extreme situation, of course, but an experimentally well defined
situation.

Sokoloff: Some of the data that you showed can be explained by failing of the
sodium-potassium pump. The sodium-potassium pump depends not only on sodium and
potassium, the concentrations of which should be at the right levels, but it is a
membrane enzyme which is dependant on other compounds which are in the membrane,
in particular, phospholipids. Some of those phospholipids turn over fairly rapidly,
and I was wondering if you thought about examining phospholipids in the lesion?

Hossmann: We did not measure phospholipids, but this brings us to the question of
free radical reactions. Dr. Zalewska from Warszaw measured antioxidants in infarcted territory and there was in fact, a decrease as in report of Demopoulos. It is,
therefore, not unlikely that peroxidation of phospholipids occurs in the ischemic
territory.

Andjus: Hibernating animals have a different membrane and they tolerate lower
temperatures and the reason for that, from the biological point of view, is that
they have to tolerate lower temperatures during hibernation because their body
temperature is close to that of the surrounding. These animals are much more resistant
to hypoxia. There might be something in their membrane also, that helps the ATPase
to work under hypoxic conditions.

Mandel: Let's go to the problems of methodology.

Ostrowski: A general question concerning autoradiography of radioactive labelled compounds to get an idea of the distribution in the brain. Is it useful to do that generally, when I can't decide is the compound now in blood or in the brain tissue areas?

Sokoloff: It's in the brain tissue because we give a pulse in 0 time and then we allow plasma to be cleared of deoxyglucose.

Ostrowski: I don't mean deoxyglucose, I mean other radiolabelled drugs.

Sokoloff: It depends on the substance and what happens to it in the plasma and how difficult it is to get the substance across the blood brain barrier.

Ostrowski: But I am right: I can't decide by autoradiography alone if it is going through the blood brain barrier.

Sokoloff: No, you can't.

Mandel: I want to ask you a question of a man who has not to his disposal the US public health department with all your computers. Actually, you have a possibility to have a general view what is happening in the whole brain. There are some people who would be already happy if they could know what is happening in a specific area of the brain. Would it be possible with available radioactivity to measure simply the ^{14}C-deoxyglucose in the vasodilation area?

Sokoloff: Yes, some people are doing that. They do a punch biopsy and then measure radioactivity in the tissue.

Mandel: Is there no radioactivity in the situation in which it could be measured at least about 40 minutes after administration?

Sokoloff: Yes, there is in the normal rat, for example between 4 and 10 mμCi/g.

Mandel: So it will be possible.

Hoyer: I would like to come back to the deoxyglucose method and its use in patients. You showed it in your last slide. As we know, we have no similar decrease in blood flow and in metabolic brain parameter in dementia patients. There are dissocations between these three values, that means we should measure all these three parameters to get a good knowledge on these disturbances. If we should measure these parameters, we should use the methods, one after the other, that means for half an hour blood flow, for half an hour the CMR oxygen and perhaps for half an hour CMR glucose, that would mean that it is very difficult to keep a steady state in one dementia patient over a period of let me say 1 - 2 hours. Would it be possible to concentrate these three measurements into one, that means that we can measure blood flow by inhalation and CMR O_2 by inhalation and deoxyglucose by intravenous application of a bolus at the same time? I think this would be of great importance in patients.

Sokoloff: This is under development and there are already some results that look promising. By using oxygen to measure oxygen consumption and from the clearance of the radioactive water that is formed to measure blood flow, both blood flow

and oxygen consumption may be measured at the same time. The model has not been
completely developed. There are still problems. But I think enough has been done
to make it look like it is possible to develop a suitable model to measure blood
flow and oxygen consumption at the same time.

Mandel: To adapt the enthusiasm to the possibility: I would like to ask Dr. Sokoloff a question: How many equipments do exist now in the world?

Sokoloff: There is one in Brookhaven, one in Philadelphia, one in Saint Louis,
one in Los Angeles, one in London, one being installed in N.I.H. and six have
been approved.

Mandel: Is it extremely expensive?

Sokoloff: The one that the N.I.H. purchased was 380.000 US Dollars.

Krieglstein: I have a special question to Dr. Sokoloff: We now know something
about the intracellular distribution of hexokinase and we know that hexokinase is
bound to the mitochondria and is present in a soluble form. Main regulator of this
distribution of hexokinase is glucose-6-phosphate. Perhaps also deoxy-glucose-6-
phosphate. Do you think that the enhancement of deoxy-glucose-6-phosphate in the
brain with your method, may influence this distribution?

Sokoloff: Yes, I think it has been demonstrated that the energy metabolism will
affect the distribution of bound and free hexokinase. Although the bound and free
hexokinase have different kinetic properties the difference is not with the
hexoses. So it does not affect lump constant.

Mandel: We have one minute more to discuss the problems of therapy, all concerning the available therapy, the proposed therapy and the science fiction
therapy or we can come back to that in the afternoon. Thank you.

The Role of Sympathetic Innervation in the Regulation of Cerebral Blood Flow During Hypercapnia

O. Hudlicka* and C. T. Hing**

*Department of Physiology, Medical School, University of
Birmingham, Birmingham, UK
**Department of Bioengineering, University of California,
San Diego, La Jolla, California 92093, USA

ABSTRACT

The involvement of adrenergic and cholinergic nerves in the modulation of the
increase in cerebral blood flow during hypercapnia is a matter of controversy. It
is supposed that cholinergic fibres initiate it while adrenergic fibres have either
no effect or limit it. We have shown, using hydrogen clearance to measure cortical
blood flow in rabbits, that the cholinergically mediated component of hypercapnic
vasodilatation is completely eliminated by acute bilateral extirpation of the
superior cervical sympathetic ganglia. This presents an evidence for the opposing
effect of sympathetic cholinergic and adrenergic fibres during metabolic vasodilatation of cerebral vessels.

Chronic sympathectomy increased the hypercapnic increase in cortical blood flow.
It also increased the dilatation of small pial arteries to acid and the constriction in response to alkaline mock cerebrospinal fluid. It is therefore suggested
that sympathetic adrenergic nerve fibres limit excessive metabolic vasodilatation
and vasoconstriction which might be important in severe hyper- and hypocapnia.

KEYWORDS

Sympathetic cholinergic fibres; adrenergic nerve fibres; cortical blood flow; pial
arteries; hypercapnia; hypocapnia.

INTRODUCTION

Morphological evidence for adrenergic innervation of cerebral blood vessels is,
after many studies with Falck-Hillarp's fluorescence technique, beyond any dispute
(e.g. Falck, Mchedlishvili & Owman, 1965; Nielsen & Owman, 1967; Edvinsson, 1975;
Owman & Edvinsson, 1977). Cholinergic innervation was demonstrated by Chorobski
& Penfield (1932), and confirmed in later studies using histochemical techniques
and electron microscopy (e.g. Iwayama, Furness & Burnstock, 1970; Edvinsson, Falck
& Owman, 1977; Owman & Edvinsson, 1977). However, the role of both adrenergic and
cholinergic innervation in the regulation of cerebral blood flow is still obscure
- probably due to the lack of suitable techniques or animal models.

It was suggested that the nervous system might be involved in the modulation of
the response of cerebral blood vessels to changes in arterial pCO_2. Greenberg,
Reivich & Noordergraaf (1978) assumed an involvement of a nervous component in the

increase in cerebral blood flow during hypercapnia since the onset of vasodilatation was considerably faster in the experimental situation than the predicted speed
of onset determined by modelling the cerebral blood flow (CBF) response using
measured values of pCO_2, pH and bicarbonate in the blood and cerebrospinal fluid
(CSF).   Rovere and others (1973) and Scremin, Rubinstein & Sonnenschein (1977,
1978) found that the increase in cortical blood flow during hypercapnia could be
blocked by atropine and potentiated by eserine.   They therefore assumed that the
response involved a cholinergic component.   However, Hoff, McKenzie & Harper
(1977) could not alter this response by either uni- or bilateral section of the
7th cranial nerve which is supposed to be the main supply of cholinergic fibres
to brain vessels (Ponte & Purves, 1974; Edvinsson & Owman, 1975).   Kawamura and
others (1975), on the basis of their experiments in which atropine blocked the
response to hypercapnia when applied intracisternally, but not intravenously,
suggested that cholinergic neurons located in the brain stem were involved in this
response.   Such evidence indicates that the cholinergic innervation of cerebral
blood vessels may be from sympathetic nerves as suggested by Iwayama, Furness &
Burnstock (1970) on the basis of electronmicroscopic evidence for both adrenergic
and cholinergic nerve endings in the anterior cerebral artery in rats.   Our experiments were therefore designed to examine the part played by both types of innervation in the increase in CBF during hypercapnia.

Involvement of adrenergic sympathetic fibres in the response of cerebral blood
vessels during hypercapnia was suggested by Harper and others (1972) who found
greater effect of sympathetic stimulation in hypercapnia than in normocapnia.
Rosenblum & Commonwealth (1977) found maximal response of pial arteries to sympathetic stimulation at relatively low pH of CSF.   Both these findings would suggest
that activation of adrenergic nerve fibres would limit metabolic vasodilatation,
and, consequently, such vasodilatation should be more pronounced in sympathectomised animals.   To test this hypothesis we examined changes in cortical blood flow
during hypercapnia, and changes in the diameter of pial arteries in CSF of different compositions in acutely or chronically sympathectomised animals.

Finally we tried to find out whether the absence of sympathetic innervation would
modify the reactivity of pial arteries in conscious animals under circumstances
when their cardiovascular system, particularly the cerebral circulation, would be
exposed to a cardiovascular stress.   Such a stress can be achieved in rabbits by
placing them into the vertical position (Meessen & Schmidt, 1943).

METHODS

All experiments were performed on New Zealand Red or White rabbits 2-4 kg body
weight.   Care was taken to select animals with no admixture of black colour since
the presence of atropinase is linked to the gene for black colour (Kalow, 1962).
Experiments were performed under pentobarbitone anaesthesia 30 mg/kg i.v., supple-
mented as necessary to maintain it at a level when the corneal reflex would be
present without any limb movements.   Blood pressure was measured in a cannula
inserted into one femoral artery.   The femoral vein was cannulated for i.v. inject-
ions, and the trachea was also cannulated.   Cortical blood flow in the frontal and
parietal region was measured by the hydrogen clearance method (Aukland, Bower &
Berliner, 1964), using platinum electrodes of about 80 μm diameter, inserted up to
1.8 mm into the cortex.   An indifferent silver-silver chloride electrode was placed
under the skin in the neck.   Pure hydrogen was given into the tracheal cannula for
not more than 2 min through a 18 gauge needle at a pressure which made the stream
of the gas just palpable.   During this period, arterial pCO_2 and pH did not change
but pO_2 decreased by as much as 40 mmHg.   However, all values were back to control
within one minute after the end of hydrogen inhalation.

A hydrogen clearance curve was evaluated during 10 min following hydrogen inhalation, discarding readings during the first minute when arterial pO_2 was returning to control values. Hypercapnia was induced by breathing 5% CO_2 in air for 2 min; this produced a rise in $paCO_2$ from 24.6 ± 1.7 mmHg to 31.9 ± 1.7 mmHg and a fall in pH from 7.416 ± 0.01 to 7.373 ± 0.02. Atropine (0.4-0.6 mg/kg) was given intravenously.

Sympathectomy was performed by bilateral extirpation of superior cervical ganglia and in the case of chronic sympathectomy this was done under halothane anaesthesia and with aseptic conditions two days before the experiments.

In experiments on pial arteries, observations were made through a cranial window sealed into a hole in the skull and covered with a glass cover slip. Two holes in the wall of the window fitted with polyethylene tubing enabled perfusion with mock cerebrospinal fluid of different compositions (3.0 mM KCl, 2.4 mM $MgCl_2$, 5.0 mM $CaCl_2$, 3.7 mM glucose, 6.0 mM urea, and NaCl varying from 139 mM in combination with 11 mM $NaHCO_3$ to 150 mM with no bicarbonate or 125 mM with 25 mM bicarbonate). The solutions were bubbled with 5% CO_2 in 95% N_2 to ensure a stable pCO_2 in any particular experiment with a variation between 15-25 mmHg in different experiments. They were kept under a thick layer of liquid paraffin at $37^{\circ}C$. pH varied between 6.56-7.006 in solutions without bicarbonate, from 7.287-7.497 in control solutions and from 7.558-7.768 in solutions with 25 mM bicarbonate in different experiments. The diameter of pial arteries was measured by a scale in the eye piece.

In experiments on conscious animals, diameters of pial vessels were measured from enlarged photographs. Systolic blood pressure was measured indirectly from ear arteries (Grant & Rotschild, 1934). All values are expressed as mean ± S.E. Student's unpaired t-test was used for statistical analysis.

    RESULTS

Cortical blood flow at rest was 49.3 ± 3.1 ml/100g.min in the right frontal cortex, and 55.2 ± 2.2 ml/100g.min in the right parietal cortex. We found, in agreement with the results of Rovere and others (1973) and Scremin, Rubinstein & Sonnenschein (1977, 1978) that the increase in blood flow during inhalation of 5% CO_2, which was 21.9 ± 1.9% in the frontal and 23.9 ± 2% in the parietal cortex, could be almost abolished by administration of atropine (Fig. 1). If, however, animals were bilaterally sympathectomised, either acutely or chronically, the response to CO_2 was not affected by atropine. The increase in blood flow in response to 5% CO_2 inhalation in acutely sympathectomised animals was similar to that in intact animals, and slightly greater in chronically sympathectomised animals. These results suggest that atropine was blocking the effect of cholinergic nerve fibres which travel to the cerebral blood vessels through the superior cervical ganglia.

In contrast, acute sympathectomy did not affect the response to hypercapnia in animals without atropine while chronic sympathectomy produced a significantly greater increase in blood flow (Fig. 2) this being more so in the frontal than in the parietal region. This would indicate that adrenergic nerve fibres limited the cholinergically mediated hypercapnic increase in CBF. Chronic sympathectomy probably increased the sensitivity of cortical vessels to carbon dioxide, or rather to the changes in pH in the CSF.

Similar results were obtained from observations of the pial vessels. As expected, the greatest response to either acid or alkaline mock CSF was seen in the smallest arteries (inner diameter 50-100 μm). Arteries 100-200 μm dilated or constricted less, and arteries > 200 μm less still. When the diameter of arteries in 11 mM

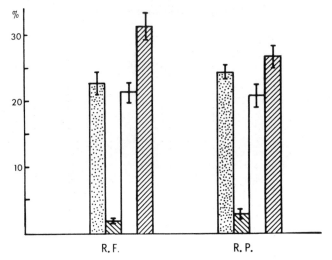

Fig. 1.   Changes in rabbit cortical blood flow measured by
          hydrogen clearance method during 2 min inhalation
          of 5% CO_2 in a control period (▨), after atropine
          (▨), and in acutely (☐) and chronically
          (▨) sympathectomised and atropinized animals
          breathing 5% CO_2. RF = right frontal cortex, RP =
          right parietal cortex. Means ± S.E.

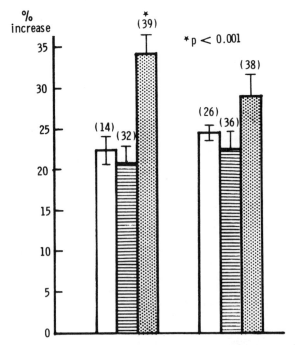

Fig. 2.   Changes in cortical blood flow in control (☐),
          acutely (▤) and chronically (▨) sympathect-
          omised animals breathing 5% CO_2. Means ± S.E.
          Number of measurements in parenthesis.

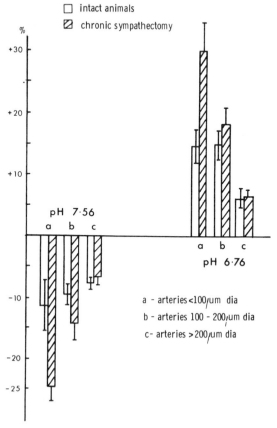

CHANGES IN PARIETAL PIAL VESSELS DIAMETERS
WITH DIFFERENT pH OF CSF

☐ intact animals
▨ chronic sympathectomy

Fig. 3.   Changes in the diameters of arteries in pial vessels
          in rabbit parietal cortex in response to solutions
          with different concentrations of HCO_3^- (25 mM and 0)
          expressed as % of the diameters in 11 mM HCO_3. a =
          arteries < 100 μm, b = arteries 100-200 μm, c =
          arteries > 200 μm, control animals, chronically
          sympathectomised animals. Means ± S.E. Number of
          measurements in parenthesis.

bicarbonate was taken as the control, the smallest arteries dilated by 14.5% in
mock CSF without bicarbonate when innervated, by 29.2% when acutely denervated
and by 30.0% when chronically denervated. Chronic denervation also produced a
greater constriction in response to 25 mM bicarbonate (Fig. 3). Reactivity of
larger arteries was not affected by either acute or chronic sympathectomy.

These findings indicate that the presence of the adrenergic sympathetic innervation is important in limiting metabolic vasodilatation produced by hypercapnia or
metabolic constriction produced by hypocapnia due e.g. to hyperventilation. This
assumption was tested in conscious rabbits exposed to orthostatic collapse.

Observations were made on pial arteries of 100–150 μm. When the animals were
brought from horizontal to vertical position, the rate of respiration increased
from 90 to 120/min. BP decreased from 125 mmHg to 68 mmHg and there was a marked
vasoconstriction in the skin. The diameters of pial arteries decreased to about
80% of control value after 10 min in the vertical position, and did not significantly change until the full development of orthostatic collapse. Collapse was
characterised by a brief apnoea and disappearance of corneal reflexes. During
restitution, respiration rate increased up to 160 per min, blood pressure returned
to control values within 20 min and the diameter of pial arteries increased (Fig.
4). Sympathectomised animals had similar symptoms as controls, similar initial
blood pressure (135 mmHg) and similar changes in the diameter of pial arteries
during the first 10 min in vertical position and during the orthostatic collapse.
However, while the control rabbits could sustain a vertical position for up to
75 min, collapse in sympathectomised animals developed after 22 min in spite of a
smaller decrease in blood pressure. During 20 min restitution, blood pressure
returned to control values, but the diameter of pial arteries significantly
decreased. Recovery of sympathectomised animals took considerably longer than
that of control animals, and some of the rabbits did not recover at all.

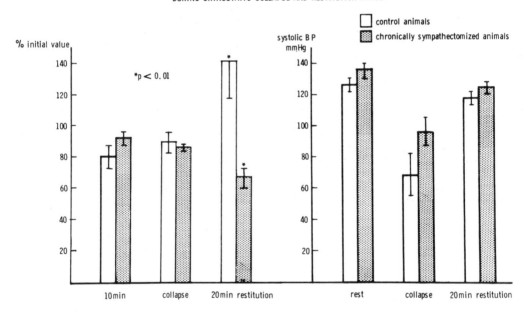

Fig. 4.   Changes in the diameters of pial arteries (left side)
           and systolic blood pressure in mmHg (right side) in
           control and chronically sympathectomised animals.
           Diameters at 10 min in vertical position, during
           orthostatic collapse and at 20 min of restitution
           after collapse expressed as % of resting values (=
           100%). Experiments on 5 control and 6 sympathectom-
           ised animals.

DISCUSSION

The main findings presented here show that

a) Increase in cortical blood flow during hypercapnia which can be blocked by
    atropine is mediated by fibres passing through or originating in the
    superior cervical ganglion.

b) Acute sympathectomy which eliminates both cholinergic and adrenergic fibres,
    brings this response back to normal.

c) Chronic sympathectomy increases the cortical vasodilatation in response to
    hypercapnia and sensitivity of small pial arteries to vasodilatation and
    vasoconstriction in response to changes in pH of the CSF.

Both findings are rather unexpected. Firstly, there is no morphological evidence
of cholinergic pathways from the superior cervical ganglion. Iwayama, Furness &
Burnstock (1970) who found cholinergic and adrenergic nerve endings of sympathetic
origin in the rat claimed that they were not coming from the superior cervical
ganglion. Plechkova and others (1969) and Peerless & Yasargil (1971) described
cholinergic fibres accompanying adrenergic in pial vessels in rabbits, but none
of these authors mention their origin. Edvinsson (1975) found the highest density
of cholinergic fibres around the internal carotid and middle cerebral artery in
cats but again could not trace their origin - they did not degenerate either
after the section of the intracranial part of cranial nerves or after superior
cervical gangliectomy.

It might be possible that rabbit has a different pathway for cholinergic fibres
than either the rat or the cat, but this possibility needs further experimental
study. However, it is quite clear that these cholinergic fibres are involved in
the hypercapnic increase in CBF since atropine can no longer affect it when the
nerves are acutely sectioned.

The role of adrenergic fibres in the modulation of hypercapnic vasodilatation
seems to be somewhat more complicated. Acute sympathectomy was without any
effect. This is in agreement with the experiments of Traystman & Rapela (1975)
who found no effect of sympathetic nerves on the increase in CBF during hypercapnia, but seemingly contrary to the findings of Kawamura and others (1974) who
found an enhanced response to hypercapnia after phenoxybenzamine in baboons. Acid
pH is known to inhibit uptake of noradrenaline (Edvinsson & Owman, 1977) and to
enhance the effect of adrenergic stimuli on pial arteries (Rosenblum & Commonwealth,
1977). This results in a limiting effect of adrenergic fibres on metabolic vasodilatation as seen in our experiments with atropine: while the adrenergic fibres
were intact and cholinergic eliminated, the hypercapnic increase in blood flow was
very much reduced. When the adrenergic as well as cholinergic fibres were eliminated by acute sympathectomy, the response to hypercapnia was similar as with both
types of fibres intact. It thus appears that the tone of cortical arteries is a
result of the balanced effect of both cholinergic and adrenergic fibres.

The reasons for a larger increase in cortical blood flow in response to hypercapnia
in chronically sympathectomised animals might be due to the fact that at this stage
the vessels became more sensitive to different changes in the ion concentration
which would affect Ca^{++} entry into the vascular smooth muscle. This seems to affect
 most smaller pial arterioles which are normally more sensitive to changes in
hydrogen ion concentrations than larger ones. Both dilatation in response to acid
and constriction in response to alkaline mock CSF were significantly greater in
chronically sympathectomised animals than in acutely denervated, indicating that,
as long as the adrenergic nerve fibres are not degenerated, they might restrict
metabolic vasodilatation or constriction. This effect was particularly obvious if

constriction of pial arteries was produced by hypercapnia in conscious animals in
the model of orthostatic collapse. In these experiments the role of sympathetic
nerve fibres innervating brain vessels was so essential that it increased greatly
the resistance towards the collapse and improved the chances of survival. This
model can thus serve well to investigate the role of sympathetic nervous system
in the regulation of cerebral blood flow.

REFERENCES

Aukland, K., B. F. Bower, and R. W. Berliner (1964). Measurement of local blood
    flow with hydrogen gas. Circ. Res., 14, 164-187.
Chorobski, J., and W. Penfield (1932). Cerebral vasodilator nerves and their
    pathway from the medulla oblongata with observations of the pial and intra-
    cerebral vascular plexus. Archs Neurol. Psychiat., 28, 1257-1289.
Edvinsson, L. (1975). Neurogenic mechanisms in the cerebrovascular bed. Acta
    physiol. scand. suppl., 427, 5-35.
Edvinsson, L., B. Falck, and Ch. Owman (1977). Possibilities for a cholinergic
    action on smooth musculature and on sympathetic axons in brain vessels
    mediated by muscarinic and nicotinic receptors. J. Pharmacol. Exper. Therap.,
    200, 117-126.
Edvinsson, L., and Ch. Owman (1975). Pharmacological identification of adrenergic
    (alpha and beta), cholinergic (muscarinic and nicotinic), histaminergic (H_1
    and H_2) and serotonergic receptors in isolated intra and extracranial vessels.
    In M. Harper, B. Jennett, D. Miller, and J. Rowan (Eds.), Blood Flow and
    Metabolism in the Brain. Churchill Livingstone. pp. 18-25.
Edvinsson, L., and Ch. Owman (1977). Characterisation of the uptake of ^{3}H nor-
    adrenaline into rabbit brain vessels and its relation to the degree of
    sympathetic nerve supply. In Neurogenic Control of the Brain Circulation.
    Pergamon Press. pp. 121-132.
Falck, B., G. I. Mchedlishvili, and Ch. Owman (1965). Histochemical demonstration
    of adrenergic nerves in cortex-pia of rabbit. Acta pharmac. tox., 23, 133-142.
Grant, R. T., and P. Rotschild (1934). A device for estimating blood pressure in
    the rabbit. J. Physiol., 81, 265-269.
Greenberg, J. H., M. Reivich, and A. Noordergraaf (1978). A model of cerebral
    blood flow in hypercapnia. Am. Biomed. Eng., 6, 453-491.
Harper, A. M., V. D. Deshmukh, J. O. Rowan, and W. B. Jennett (1972). The
    influence of sympathetic nervous activity on cerebral blood flow. Arch.
    neurol., 27, 1-6.
Hoff, J. T., E. T. McKenzie, and A. M. Harper (1977). Responses of the cerebral
    circulation to hypercapnia and hypoxia after 7th cranial nerve transection in
    baboons. Circ. Res., 40, 258-262.
Iwayama, T., J. B. Furness, and G. Burnstock (1970). Dual adrenergic and cholin-
    ergic innervation of the cerebral arteries of the rat. Circ. Res., 26, 635-
    646.
Kalow, W. (1962). Pharmacogenetics, Heredity and the Response to Drugs. W. B.
    Saunders Company, Philadelphia London. pp. 53-56.
Kawamura, Y., J. S. Meyer, H. Hiromoto, M. Aoyagi, and K. Hashi (1974). Myogenic
    control of cerebral blood flow in the baboon. Effects of alpha adrenergic
    blockade with phenoxybenzamine on cerebral autoregulation and vasomotor
    reactivity to changes in $paCO_2$. Stroke, 5, 747-758.
Kawamura, Y., J. S. Meyer, H. Hiromoto, M. Aoyagi, Y. Tagashira, and E. O. Ott
    (1975). Neurogenic control of cerebral blood flow in the baboon. Effect of
    the cholinergic inhibitory agent, atropine, on cerebral autoregulation and
    vasomotor reactivity to changes in $paCO_2$. J. Neurosurg., 43, 676-688.
Meessen, H., and R. Schmidt (1943). Uber Durchblutungstorungen der Netzhautgefasse
    bei exp. Kollaps. Arch. Kreislaufforsch., 10, 8-15.

Nielsen, K. C., and Ch. Owman (1967). Adrenergic innervation of pial arteries related to the circle of Willis in the cat. Brain Res., 6, 773-776.

Owman, Ch., and L. Edvinsson (1977). Neurogenic control of brain circulation. Pergamon Press.

Peerless, S. J., and M. G. Yasargil (1971). Adrenergic innervation of the cerebral blood vessels in the rabbit. J. Neurosurg., 35, 148-154.

Plechkova, E. K., G. I. Mchedlishvili, N. B. Lavrentyeva, and L. C. Nikolayshvili (1969). Cholinergic·mechanism involved in the functional dilatation of cortical cerebral arteries (in Russian). In Correlation of Blood Supply with Metabolism and Function. G. Mchedlishvili (Ed.). Publishing House Metsniereba, Tbilishi. pp. 172-178.

Ponte, J., and M. J. Purves (1974). The role of the carotid body chemoreceptors and carotid sinus baroreceptors in the control of cerebral blood vessels. J. Physiol., 237, 315-340.

Rosenblum, W. I., and V. Commonwealth (1977). Vascular resistance in the cerebral circulation: location and potential consequences with respect to the effect of neurogenic stimuli on flow. In Ch. Owman, and L. Edvinsson (Eds.), Neurogenic Control of the Brain Circulation. Pergamon Press. pp. 221-229.

Rovere, A. A., O. V. Scremin, M. R. Beresi, A. C. Raynald, and A. Giardini (1973). Cholinergic mechanism in the cerebrovascular action of carbon dioxide. Stroke, 4, 969-972.

Scremin, O. V., E. H. Rubinstein, and R. R. Sonnenschein (1977). Cholinergic modulation of the cerebrovascular response to CO_2 in the rabbit. In Ch. Owman, and L. Edvinsson (Eds.), Neurogenic Control of the Brain Circulation. Oxford, Pergamon. pp. 471-481.

Scremin, O. V., E. H. Rubinstein, and R. R. Sonnenschein (1978). Cerebrovascular CO_2 reactivity: role of a cholinergic mechanism modulated by anaesthesia. Stroke, 9, 160-165.

Traystman, R. J., and C. E. Rapela (1975). Effect of sympathetic nerve stimulation on cerebral and cephalic blood flow in dogs. Circ. Res., 36, 620-630.

This work was supported by a grant from the British Medical Research Council.

DISCUSSION

Sokoloff: Thank you very much for your interesting paper. It's open for discussion. In the explanation you offered for the results, you conclude that under normal circumstances the adrenergic supply is not doing anything special and not a chronic effect.

Hudlicka: That is correct. I think that the adrenergic supply is really doing something under extreme circumstances.

Sokoloff: So that in many experiments when people have done cerebral sympathectomy and found that it didn't change cerebral blood flow, this can be compatible to your results.

Hudlicka: Yes, but it is compatible with our results, because I think, that if you are doing it under resting conditions, you can't expect much.

Hossmann: I have two questions: You demonstrated an increase in blood flow during hypercapnia with 5 % CO_2 by about 20 %. Why this is so low.

Hudlicka: We did not let the animals to breath carbon dioxide for to long so it was a very mild hypercapnia, and the p CO_2 only increased from 25 to 32 mm Hg.

Hossmann: The other question I have: after shock or after recovery from shock one would expect reactive hyperemia, and during reactive hyperemia, the vessels do not react to CO_2. In the sympathectomized animals the blood pressure decrease during the rise in vertical position was not so extensive as in the normal intact animals. And therefore I would expect that in the sympathectomized animals, the cerebral ischemia was less pronounced than in the intact animals, that reactive hyperemia was shorter and a recovery of CO_2 reactivity more rapid.

Hudlicka: The fact is that in the sympathectomized animals, there was never ever any reactive hyperemia as judged by the diameters of pial arteries.

Hossmann: Even at shorter intervals not?

Hudlicka: That's right.

Martorana: After sympathectomy, you have an increased sensitivity. What is inducing it? Circulating catecholamines, perhaps?

Hudlicka: That's a very good question of which I would like to know the answer. It might be supersensitivity to noradrenaline. But sympathectomy may effect many different factors which could influence the entry of calcium into the vascular smooth muscle and which could probably change the sensitivity.

Sokoloff: Several years ago, John Pickard from Glasgow published the very provocative paper in "Nature New Biology" in which he reported that the administration of Indomethacine, which blocks the synthesis of prostaglandines, also blocks the carbon dioxide vasodilation of cerebral vessels, and I have not heard anymore about this since.

Hudlicka: Neither have I. I am familiar with this paper.

Chronic Normobaric Hypoxia and Subcellular Isoenzyme Patterns of Rat Brain Lactate Dehydrogenase

H. H. Berlet*, V. Stefanovich**, B. Volk***, T. Lehnert*
and M. Franz*

*Institute of Pathochemistry and General Neurochemistry,
University Centre of Pathology, Heidelberg,
Federal Republic of Germany
**Hoechst AG Werk Albert, Wiesbaden-Biebrich, Federal
Republic of Germany
***Institute of Neuropathology, University Centre of Pathology,
Heidelberg, Federal Republic of Germany

ABSTRACT

In rats exposed to normobaric hypoxia (10 % O_2) for seven days, soluble and bound lactate dehydrogenase (LDH) activity of subcellular fractions of brain including synaptosomes, free mitochondria, microsomes and myelin was determined as well as the respective isoenzyme patterns. Additional 'latent' enzyme activity was measured in samples incubated with Triton X-100. Hypoxia resulted in an apparently compensated mild state of respiratory alkalosis and a markedly reduced oxygen saturation of blood. The cerebral energy state showed little deviation from normal, except for a slight decrease of ATP and a significant increase of lactate levels. In the absence of gross changes in apparent enzyme activity we observed marked decreases of the bound 'latent' activity. Electrophoretically, there was a general tendency of LDH-1 and other anodal isoenzymes to rise. Thus, chronic hypoxia did entail changes of LDH regarding both its subcellular distribution and individual molecular forms, possibly of an adaptive nature.

KEYWORDS

Chronic hypoxia; rats; brain; lactate dehydrogenase activity; lactate dehydrogenase isoenzymes; subcellular distribution; latent enzyme activity; Triton X-100; electron microscopy.

INTRODUCTION

Levels of high-energy compounds and related metabolites are commonly used to assess the metabolic state of tissues in acute experiments. In chronic experiments, a seemingly normal steady state may develop as a result of adaptation through some form of enzyme regulation at the cellular level. In this context the possible significance of so-called 'ambiquitous' enzymes (Wilson, 1978) has emerged from studies on the reversible binding of glycolytic enzymes including hexokinase and aldolase to intracellular membrane surfaces (Masters, 1978; Masters, Sheedy and Winzor, 1969).
Recent studies in our laboratory have shown that LDH may also belong to this group of enzymes. Substantial enzyme activities were found to be associated with particle fragments of rat brain homogenates, and additional activity became measurable when the particle fragments were treated with a mild detergent (Berlet and Lehnert, 1978).

75

Furthermore differential isoenzyme patterns of LDH suggested a relationship of the
enzyme to a complex subcellular metabolic compartmentation. The present study is
dealing with the effects of mild chronic hypoxia in rats on some of these features
of LDH in rat brain to find out how LDH isoenzymes might be involved in the metabolic adaptation of brain tissue to hypoxia.

MATERIALS AND METHODS

Male Wistar rats weighing 180 to 220 g were kept for seven days in a special chamber aerated with a mixture of 10 % O_2 and 90 % N_2. The experimental atmosphere was
continously monitored for its oxygen content, temperature and humidity, and for
CO_2 at regular intervals. The animals were allowed free access to food and water.
Control animals were maintained in a normal atmosphere but under otherwise identical conditions. Native brain for enzyme studies was obtained from unanesthetized
animals removed from the chamber and at once decapitated. Frozen brain tissue for
the analysis of labile compounds was collected by means of a brain blowing device
installed inside the chamber (Veech and co-workers, 1973), and blood for the measurements of pH and blood gases was drawn from the abdominal aorta of halothane-
anesthetized animals. Animals for electron microscopic examinations were anesthetized with nembutal inside the chamber and taken out for immediate perfusion
through the lower abdominal aorta with Rheomacrodex followed by 0.14 M glutaraldehyde. Samples of brain, spinal cord and spinal ganglia were removed and separate tissue samples from the parietal cortex, cerebellum (folia VIII), hippocampus,
hypothalamus and spinal cord were postfixed in 1 % OsO_4, dehydrated and embedded
in Araldite. Semi-thin sections were stained with toluidine blue, thin sections
with uranyl acetate and lead citrate and examined by means of a Zeiss 9A electron
microscope.

ATP, ADP, AMP, pyruvate and lactate of deep-frozen brain tissue were determined
enzymatically according to McMillan and Siesjö (1972). Blood pH and blood gases
were measured using a blood gas analyser AVL AS, automatic gas check 940. Native
whole brain was homogenized at once in 0.32 mol/l sucrose buffered with 2.5 mmol/l
tris-HCL and containing 1 mmol/l EDTA as described elsewhere (Berlet and Lehnert,
1978), and separated into particle-free cytoplasm and enriched fractions of
myelin, synaptosomes, free mitochondria and microsomes by differential and iso-
pycnic centrifugation (Gray and Whittaker, 1962). The isolated particle fractions
were washed once in isotonic sucrose and the washed pellets were resuspended in
2.5 mmol/l tris buffer and treated with three 10-second bursts of sonication
delivered through the microtip of a Branson sonifier B-12 (output 50 W). Subsequent high speed centrifugation yielded the respective subcellular soluble ex-
tracts and particulate fractions. The assay of LDH activity and isoenzyme electrophoresis were described previously (Berlet and Lehnert, 1978; Lehnert and Berlet,
1979), except for the use of a mixture of 0.6 % agar and 0.1 % agar rather than 1 %
agar for electrophoresis. Latent LDH activity was determined following the incubation of one vol. of sample with 10 vol. of a 1 % solution of Triton X-100 in
2.5 mmol/l tris buffer at 25 °C for one hour. Protein was assayed by the method
of Lowry and co-workers (1951).

RESULTS

The auxiliary measurements in blood and brain indicated that the animals were well
adapted to the moderate chronic hypoxia they lived in for seven days. In blood
pO_2 was markedly reduced while the moderate degree of hypocapnia and a slightly
more alkaline pH are evidence of a compensated state of respiratory alkalosis
(Table 1). In brain, hypoxemia hardly affected levels of ATP and the other adenine
nucleotides, and lactate showed a moderate increase only (Table 2).

TABLE 1   Blood pH and Blood Gas Measurements in Hypoxic Rats

	pH	pCO$_2$ mm Hg	pO$_2$ mm Hg
Control	7.420 + 0.030	34.1 + 4.1	96.9 + 9.1
Hypoxia	7.456 + 0.194	25.37 + 2.88	28.03 + 1.48

Results are means + SD of six animals.

TABLE 2   Cerebral Energy State of Hypoxic Rats

	ATP	ADP	AMP	Pyruvate	Lactate
Control	2.40 +0.27	0.57 +0.03	0.053 +0.020	0.097 +0.006	1.242 +0.067
Hypoxia	2.25 +0.12	0.51 +0.05	0.050 +0.010	0.093 +0.010	1.805 +0.166

Values are expressed as μmol/g wet weight. They
are means + SD of 20 animals.

The absence of any gross structural changes on electron microscopy well fits in
with this metabolic pattern. It was only on close examination that the mitochondrial matrix sometimes appeared to be less electron dense than in the controls
suggesting the subtlest morphological changes,if any at all.

Apparent LDH activity was slightly reduced in brains of hypoxic animals (Table 3)
on account of reduced enzyme activity of cytoplasm and mitochondrial and microsomal whole fractions on the basis of unit wet weight. The overall protein content
of hypoxic brain was unchanged,although the subcellular distribution of protein
points to a differential effect of hypoxia on the protein make-up of individual
fractions. The corresponding specific activities (Table 4) serve to further demonstrate that there was a loss of protein from cytoplasm, and a dissociated loss of
protein and enzyme activity in the case of synaptosomes and microsomes. The large
fall in mitochondrial specific activity must be attributed to the increased recovery of mitochondrial protein by 50 % in hypoxic animals. Altogether,hypoxia did
not appear to affect the overall LDH activity and its apparent subcellular distribution in a relevant way.

H. H. Berlet *et al.*

TABLE 3   Subcellular Distribution of Apparent Lactate Dehydrogenase Activity of Rat Brain During Hypoxia

Fraction	Enzyme activity, U/g		Total protein, mg/g	
	Control	Hypoxia	Control	Hypoxia
Whole brain	116.7 $\pm$ 3.4	109.9* $\pm$ 3.9	120.8 $\pm$ 6.4	122.4 $\pm$ 6.3
Cytoplasm	51.4 $\pm$ 1.8	46.3* $\pm$ 3.7	26.7 $\pm$ 1.4	22.4** $\pm$ 1.2
Synaptosomes	17.3 $\pm$ 0.7	17.0 $\pm$ 2.1	27.3 $\pm$ 1.0	23.7 $\pm$ 2.7
Mitochondria	5.0 $\pm$ 0.3	4.2** $\pm$ 0.4	6.0 $\pm$ 0.3	9.2** $\pm$ 0.4
Microsomes	4.1 $\pm$ 0.2	3.8 $\pm$ 0.5	16.6 $\pm$ 1.6	13.2** $\pm$ 1.0
Myelin	1.8 $\pm$ 0.1	2.4* $\pm$ 0.3	13.0 $\pm$ 0.7	13.3 $\pm$ 1.0

Results are means $\pm$ SD of 4 experiments.

*$p < 0.05$;   **$p < 0.01$ according to Student's t-test.

Subcellular recoveries of enzyme activity were 68.2 % and
67.1 %, respectively, those of protein 74.2 % and 66.8 %.

TABLE 4   Specific Activity of Subcellular Lactate Dehydro-
          genase of Rat Brain During Hypoxia

Fraction	Specific activity, mU/mg protein	
	Control	Hypoxia
Whole brain	965 + 69	898 + 34
Cytoplasm	1 935 + 160	2 059 + 149
Synaptosomes	632 + 20	731 + 161
Mitochondria	832 + 69	458 + 24**
Microsomes	246 + 15	288 + 22**
Myelin	135 + 13	181 + 9**

Results are means + SD of 4 experiments.
*p < 0.05;   **p < 0.01 according to Student's t-test.

Subcellular recoveries of enzyme activity were 68.2 % and
67.1 %, respectively, those of protein 74.2 % and 66.8 %.

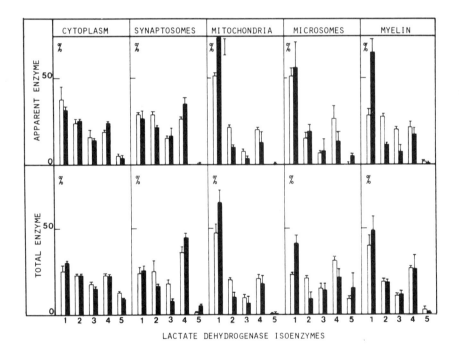

Fig. 1.   Isoenzyme patterns of soluble apparent and total i.e. deter-
          gent-treated) LDH of cytoplasm and of soluble extracts of
          subcellular fractions of rat brain during hypoxia (black co-
          lumns) compared with controls (white columns). Results are
          means + SD of four animals.

The electrophoretic studies produced clear evidence of a pronounced interaction
between chronic hypoxia and LDH of rat brain. As to <u>soluble</u> LDH (Fig. 1) hypoxia
resulted in an overall further increase of the high proportions of LDH-1 of the
particulate fractions to begin with, with some exceptions, however. Both the apparent and total LDH of synaptosomes gained in the percentages of LDH-4 and LDH-5 as
well. The basic control patterns exhibited very little LDH-5 altogether except for
the microsomal enzyme in which hypoxia caused a further increase of this molecular
form of LDH in addition to that of LDH-1. Thus the isoenzyme patterns of each of
the subcellular LDH enzymes appeared to respond to hypoxia in its own way. Some
similarity regarding their isoenzyme patterns existed between cytoplasm and
myelin although the percentage of LDH-1 of myelin was much higher than that of
cytoplasmic LDH-1. The same applies to apparent mitochondrial and microsomal LDH
but not to detergent-treated enzyme as only the proportions of microsomal LDH-5
went up.

The isoenzyme patterns of <u>bound</u> LDH (Fig. 2) were distinctly characterized by the
presence of substantial proportions of LDH-5 throughout, and they were both dissi-
milar to each other and to the respective patterns of the soluble enzyme (Fig. 1).
Similarly to soluble LDH but in a much more striking way rose the proportions of
LDH-1 of all subcellular fractions during hypoxia, accompanied by reduced proportions of LDH-5 and LDH-4. From these patterns the shift of the isoenzyme distribution from the cathodal towards the anodal isoenzymes induced by hypoxia was
even more clearly evident than from soluble LDH.

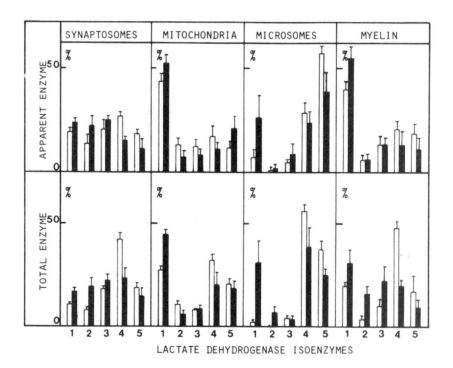

Fig. 2.   Isoenzyme patterns of <u>bound</u> apparent and total LDH of sub-
          cellular fractions of rat brain during hypoxia (black
          columns) compared with controls (white columns).
          Results are means ± SD of four animals.

TABLE 5 Latent Activity of Soluble and Bound Lactate
Dehydrogenase During Hypoxia

| Fraction | Latent activity in % of apparent activity | | | |
| | Soluble LDH | | Bound LDH | |
	Control	Hypoxia	Control	Hypoxia
Cytoplasm	7	10	–	–
Synaptosomes	19	22	45	18
Mitochondria	0	23	39	9
Microsomes	2	14	313	71
Myelin	2	27	545	149

0 not present.

Samples of the various subcellular fractions were treated with Triton X-100 (s.
methods) to measure latent LDH activity of soluble and particle-bound enzyme
(Table 5). In the controls there was only little soluble latent LDH as opposed to
bound latent enzyme activity which was markedly activated by the detergent. This
portion was drastically reduced by hypoxia and obviously converted into a soluble
latent form.

TABLE 6 'Aerobic' Subunit B of Soluble and Bound Detergent-treated Lactate Dehydrogenase in Percent[a]
During Hypoxia

| Fraction | % Soluble subunit B | | % Bound subunit B | |
	Control	Hypoxia	Control	Hypoxia
Cytoplasm	55.6 +3.1	60.8* +0.8	–	–
Synaptosomes	58.0 +3.5	52.8** +2.0	37.1 +0.5	50.1** +4.4
Mitochondria	73.6 +2.5	80.6** +3.7	48.2 +3.1	59.4** +2.6
Microsomes	59.3 +7.2	61.9 +6.4	18.3 +1.7	42.0** +7.7
Myelin	66.8 +2.1	73.2* +2.0	39.3 +4.5	59.9** +4.8

[a] % subunit A + % subunit B = 100;
Results are means + SD of 4 experiments.
*p < 0.05; **p < 0.01 for differences between control
and hypoxia according to Student's t-test.

Based on the fact that LDH isoenzymes are tetrameric proteins made up from the two
subunits A and B in known proportions (s. Wilkinson, 1970) total percentages of
the 'aerobic' subunit B were calculated from the experimental isoenzyme patterns
shown in Fig. 1 and 2 (Table 6). The values were derived from isoenzyme patterns of
detergent-treated samples only.In soluble LDH of controls, subunit B clearly pre-
vailed,while being lower than subunit A in bound LDH. Hypoxia increased the percen-

tage of subunit B of all but two fractions, namely the fluid space of synaptosomes
and microsomes. Although the data only show what was already evident from the
electrophoretic results, they serve to demonstrate more clearly,the significance
of the hypoxia-induced changes in isoenzyme distributions.

DISCUSSION

Rapid adaptive changes of cellular metabolism in response to acute hypoxia are
thought to preserve normal or near-normal cerebral levels of high-energy phosphates in experimental animals (Duffy, Nelson and Lowry, 1972; Berlet, 1976). Immediate adaption to acutely reduced oxygen tension is effected at the cellular level
through allosteric regulations of key enzymes of energy metabolism like phosphofructokinase (Passoneau and Lowry, 1964) and others. Although LDH does not belong
to this type of enzymes, cytoplasmic LDH does serve an important dual function in
anaerobic metabolism in that it helps preserve the formation of ATP by oxidizing
NADH while catalyzing the reduction of pyruvate whose oxidative utilization is
more or less impaired during hypoxia. Lactate formed under anaerobic conditions
will diffuse through cellular membranes into the plasma (Schumer, 1979). Therefore, altered amounts of enzyme protein rather than a change of its kinetic properties could underlie an adaptive response of LDH. Indeed, during high-altitude
training, LDH activity of rat brain was observed to rise, but not until the 20th
day of the experiment (Markelov and Simanovskii, 1968), whereas acute stagnant
hypoxia of 30 min duration, lowered total LDH activity of brain in adult rats
significantly (Jilêk and co-workers, 1973). Presently,seven days of moderate hypoxic hypoxia lowered total apparent LDH activity of brain, though only slightly,
while truly adaptive changes were indicated by marked reductions of latent-bound
enzyme activity. Such changes may result from reduced metabolic rates during hypoxia,while the moderate elevation of tissue lactate was not sufficient to evoke
additional enzyme activity by stimulating protein biosynthesis. An impaired protein synthesis due to a relative lack of energy supply at the transcriptional and
translational level may also have contributed. However, it would not be quite consistent with the normal levels of both ATP and total protein of whole brain.

Different molecular forms of an enzyme exhibiting differences in kinetic properties provide another means to meet varying metabolic requirements. In general, an
increase of the proportions of LDH isoenzymes containing subunit B was observed.
This observation is not consistent with the commonly held views on the relationships between particular types of metabolism and isoenzyme patterns of LDH. In
skeletal muscle the almost exclusive presence of LDH-5 is thought to be related to
a high proportion of anaerobic metabolism, and high lactate levels (Cahn and co-
workers, 1962; Fritz, 1965). A similar relationship may exist in fetal and
neonatal mammalian brain (Bonavita, Ponte and Amore, 1964). An increase in the
proportions of LDH-3 and LDH-4 in brain during high-altitude adaption of rats
lends further support to this notion (Markelov and Simanovskii, 1968). Conversely,
LDH-1 prevails in cardiac muscle in the presence of an aerobic metabolism, and
during ontogeny the adaptation of the organism to the aerobic environment generally coincides with an increase in the proportions of anodal forms as discussed
by Masters and Holmes (1972). They also pointed out the significance of cellular
metabolites for the epigenetic control of the biosynthesis of the two polypeptide
subunits A and B of lactate dehydrogenase. Cytoplasmic determinants involved in
the kinetics of lactate dehydrogenase are both the couples $NADH/NAD^+$and lactate/
pyruvate. On account of increments of the respective numerators both ratios increase during hypoxia, especially that of lactate/pyruvate, from a normal value
of about 10 to one of 30 (Siesjö and Nilsson, 1971). Thus, for cytoplasmatic pyruvate to be further reduced to lactate under the unfavourable equilibrium conditions of hypoxia, the high affinity of LDH-1 for pyruvate compared to that of
LDH-5 might be advantageous, the increased tissue levels of pyruvate being too
low as to inhibit LDH-1 (Wilkinson., 1970). The observed losses of latent-bound

enzyme activity further support the assumption of such a functional relationship. Isoenzyme studies of the gradual release of bound lactate dehydrogenase activity from brain particles by a detergent, disclosed that the bulk of bound enzyme was attributable to LDH-1 which was also the easiest and fastest of all enzyme forms to be solubilized (Berlet, Lehnert and Volk, 1978). All the data therefore suggest that lactate dehydrogenase has some features in common with the so-called ambiquitous cytosolic enzymes (Wilson, 1978).

REFERENCES

Berlet, H. H. (1976). Hypoxic survival of normoglycaemic young adult and adult mice in relation to cerebral metabolic rates. J. Neurochem., 26, 1267-1274.
Berlet, H. H. and T. Lehnert (1978). Differential isoenzyme patterns of soluble and particle-bound lactate dehydrogenase of rat brain. FEBS Lett., 91, 45-48.
Berlet, H. H., T. Lehnert and B. Volk (1978). Membrane-bound A_4 lactate dehydrogenase of rat brain and its possible relationship to anaerobic glycolysis. Proc. Europ. Soc. Neurochem., 1, 573.
Bonavita, V., F. Ponte and G. Amore (1964). Lactate dehydrogenase isoenzymes in the nervous tissue - IV. An ontogenetic study on the rat brain. J. Neurochem., 11, 39-47.
Cahn, R. D., N. O. Kaplan, L. Levine and E. Zwilling (1962). Nature and development of lactic dehydrogenases. Science, 136, 862-969.
Duffy, T. E., S. R. Nelson and O. H. Lowry (1972). Cerebral carbohydrate metabolism during acute hypoxia and recovery. J. Neurochem., 19, 959-977.
Fritz, P. J. (1965). Rabbit muscle lactate dehydrogenase 5, a regulatory enzyme. Science, 150, 364-366.
Gray, E. G. and V. P. Whittaker (1962). The isolation of nerve endings from brain: an electron microscopic study of cell fragments derived by homogenization and centrifugation. J. Anat., 96, 79-88.
Jilek, L., V. Janata, A. Londonová, Z. Makoc, S. Trojan and F. Vorel (1973). The influence of stagnant hypoxia on the activity of some dehydrogenases and aminotransferases in the brain of rats during ontogenesis. Develop. Psychobiol., 6, 139-146.
Lehnert, T. and H. H. Berlet (1979). Selective inactivation of lactate dehydrogenase of rat tissues by sodium deoxycholate. Biochem. J., 177, 813-818.
Lowry, O. H., N. J. Rosebrough, A. L. Farr and R. J. Randall (1951). Protein measurements with the Folin phenol reagent. J. Biol. Chem., 193, 265-275.
McMillan, V. and B. K. Siesjö (1972). Brain energy metabolism in hypoxemia. Scand. J. Clin. Lab. Invest., 30, 127-136.
Markelov, I. M. and L. N. Simanovskii (1968). Activity of lactate dehydrogenase and of its isoenzymes in the blood and tissues of the rat changing as a result of training to hypoxia. Dokl. Akad. Nauk SSSR, 182, 982-984.
Masters, C. J. (1978). Interactions between soluble enzymes and subcellular structure. Trends Biochem., 3, 206-208.
Masters, C. J. and R. S. Holmes (1972). Isoenzymes and ontogeny. Biol. Rev., 47, 309-361.
Masters, C. J., R. J. Sheedy and A. J. Winzor (1969). Reversible adsorption of enzymes as a possible allosteric control mechanism. Biochem. J., 112, 806-808.
Passoneau, J. V. and O. H. Lowry (1964). The role of phosphofructokinase in metabolic regulation. Advances in Enzyme Regulation, Vol. 2 Pergamon Press, New York. pp. 265-274.
Schumer, W. (1979). Cell metabolism and lactate. In H. Bossart and C. Perret (Eds.), Lactate in Acute Conditions. S. Karger, Basel. pp. 1-9.
Siesjö, B. K. and L. Nilsson (1971). The influence of arterial hypoxemia upon labile phosphates and upon extracellular lactate and pyruvate concentration in the rat brain. Scand. J. Clin. Lab. Invest., 27, 83-96.

Veech, R. L., R. L. Harris, D. Veloso and E. H. Veech (1973). Freeze-blowing: a
    new technique for the study of brain in vivo. J. Neurochem., 20, 183-188.
Wilkinson, J. H. (1970). Isoenzymes. 2nd. ed. Chapman & Hall, London.
Wilson, J. E. (1978). Ambiquitous enzymes: variation in intracellular distribu-
    tion as a regulatory mechanism. Trends Biochem., 3, 124-125.

DISCUSSION

Sokoloff: Dr. Berlet's very interesting paper is open for discussion.

Mandel: May I ask you: Did you try to dissociate the lactate dehydrogenase by changing ionic strength?

Berlet: No, we have not yet done this. We have concentrated at the time on the detergent so far.

Porsche: Can you differentiate between lactate dehydrogenase in cytoplasma and in mitochondria?

Berlet: Again I have to confess that we have not yet done this.

Andjus: These animals were studied, if I understood you correctly, 10 days after exposure.

Berlet: The animals were studied at the end of the 7th day.

Andjus: How much do you think animals were adapted to hypoxia from the tolerance point of view? Have you made any survival test?

Berlet: No. All we can say from the data on the cerebral energy state, the animals seem to be very normal.

Andjus: In this point yes. But are they adapted, can they tolerate more hypoxia than animals not exposed to this seven day treatment? Are you dealing with animals with increased resistance or not?

Berlet: We have not yet examined animals in this respect. We should do this.

Comparative Aspects of Energy Metabolism in Nonmammalian Brains Under Normoxic and Hypoxic Conditions[1]

G. Wegener

Institut für Zoologie der Universität, D-6500 Mainz,
Federal Republic of Germany

ABSTRACT

A comparative survey is given on the energy metabolism of the central nervous systems from animals of different phyla to bring into focus general features of brain metabolism, as well as adaptations to special living conditions. All brains tested so far show a continous metabolic activity which is increased during "brainwork", in such a way yielding the possibility to detect active areas. Glucose is a favoured substrate, glycolysis is present in all nervous systems likewise. Ketone bodies are alternative substrates in all brains, while the oxidation of fatty acids seems to be restricted to certain insect groups. Contrary to mammals, the lower animals have significant fuel stores. In all species the CNS is among the organs with the highest oxygen consumption. Nevertheless, in the lower animals the capacity of aerobic pathways is restricted. The insect brain, however, is highly aerobic, its oxygen consumption is the highest ever measured in nervous tissue.
The extreme vulnerability of the mammalian brain to an interruption of energy production, is a special feature. The brains of lower animals are more tolerant to conditions which easily kill mammals. It is expected that certain aspects of brain metabolism can be advantageously studied with the less sensitive nervous systems of lower animals.

KEYWORDS

Energy metabolism of CNS; comparative aspects; vertebrates and invertebrates; fuels of the brain; oxygen consumption of brains; hypoxia; anaerobic brain metabolism.

---

[1] This paper is gratefully dedicated to my teacher, Bernhard Rensch, Professor emeritus of Zoology at Münster (Westf.) on occasion of his 80th birthday

INTRODUCTION

Biology has two main objects; to derive general rules, valid for all living systems and to understand the vast variety of organisms. Both aims can only be approached on parallel streets and with permanent crosstraffic to exchange information. Obviously this holds true in a special manner for the neurobiology which has gained fundamental concepts and great progress from comparative physiology, i.e. the investigation of different animals. This includes the first observation of "bioelectricity" and later the demonstration of chemical transmission as well as the detection of the information code using the common frog; the studies of impulses and ionic fluxes in the squid axon; the evaluation of inhibition phenomena in the optic system of the horseshoe crab and the stretch receptor of the crayfish; the isolation of synaptosomes from electric organs of torpedo fish; the studies on behaviour and memory using lower animals, only to name a few examples.

Mammals are widely studied with respect to the energy metabolism of their brains, but nevertheless certain questions are unsettled and the subject of controversy. In this paper a short survey shall be given on the energy metabolism of the CNS from a comparative point of view. This attempt seems reasonable since in all groups of the animal kingdom the nervous tissue has the same function and a rather similar structure. So comparative studies are expected to bring into focus those general metabolic features of nervous systems inseparably connected with function. On the other hand they may show to what extent the brains' metabolism is able to adapt to special living conditions and given anatomical facts.

Both aspects may be of some interest for researchers who are studying mammals mainly for practical purposes, since lower animals may well yield model systems more advantageous for the study of certain problems.

Limitation of space enforces a strict concentration on only a few topics, mainly those to which we have made contributions ourselves. Some important points like transport of substrates, the blood-brain-barrier phenomena, glia-neuron interrelationships etc. are completely omitted.

CHARACTERISTIC FEATURES OF THE ENERGY METABOLISM IN MAMMALIAN BRAINS

The mammalian brain has some peculiarities with respect to its energy metabolism which are not found in this combination in any other of the large organs of the body.

Metabolic Activity and Brain Function

The human brain as a whole is continuously active and produces energy at a fairly constant and rather high rate, independent of the activity status of the object (Mc Ilwain and Bachelard, 1971). Nevertheless there is a strict connection in mammalian brains between local "brain work" and energy production as shown by a regionally increased cerebral blood flow (Ingvar and Lassen, 1975; Raichle and coworkers, 1976; Lassen, Ingvar, and Skinjøj, 1978) and an elevated uptake of substrate as demonstrated with the ingenuous ^{14}C-deoxyglucose method

(Sokoloff and coworkers, 1977; Sokoloff, 1977). These methods are being used to answer fundamental questions concerning both organization and function of nervous systems.

Fuels for Energy Production

Blood glucose is the only fuel the mammalian brain utilizes under normal conditions. A drastic lowering of the glucose level causes loss of brain function and electrical activity (Norberg and Siesjö, 1976). Function can readily be restored by injection of glucose.

The glucose is metabolized mainly via glycolysis, the contribution of the pentose-phosphate cycle is negligible in adult mammals and was estimated not to exceed 5 % in rats and monkeys (Hostetler and Landau, 1967; Hostetler and coworkers, 1970). The level of NADPH in functioning brain tissue is low, its kinetics were shown to be much slower than those of NADH (Jöbsis and coworkers, 1971). On the other hand there is a rapid conversion of glucose-C into amino acids via pyruvate and Krebs cycle intermediates (Vrba, 1962; Vrba, Gaitonde, and Richter, 1962; Cremer, 1964; Gaitonde, Marchi, and Richter, 1964; Gaitonde, Dahl, and Elliot, 1965; Shimada and coworkers, 1973). The main regulatory enzymes of glucose metabolism were identified to be hexokinase which is predominantly bound to mitochondria (Wilson, 1968; Vallejo, Marco, and Sebastian, 1970; Knull, Taylor, and Wells, 1973) and phosphofructokinase (Lowry and coworkers, 1964; Norberg and Siesjö, 1975).

In cases of metabolic emergency like starvation, the adult brains energy demand can be met to more than 50 % by an alternative substrate, the ketone bodies which are formed in the liver under these conditions (Cahill, Owen, and Morgan, 1968; Hawkins, Williamson, and Krebs, 1971; Sokoloff, 1973; Hawkins and Biebuyck, 1979).

The mammalian brain is virtually unable to take advantage of the ideal energy substrate fat in a direct manner (Scow and Chernick, 1970). This is not due to limited access, since fatty acids can readily pass the blood brain barrier (Dhopeswarkar and Mead, 1973), but due to the small enzymatic capacity (Wegener and Zebe, 1971; Wegener and Pfeifer, 1975). Even during extreme starvation the pattern of fatty acids in the brain is preserved and fatty acids are not utilized as an energy source (Joel and coworkers, 1974).

The drawback not to use fat for ATP production may well be compensated by two advantages. First, high concentrations of the cytotoxic fatty acids are avoided in brain tissue, second, the metabolism of the highly complex lipids, which are the basis of neuronal functioning, can proceed without competing catabolic enzyme activities.

Energy stores

In spite of its permanently high metabolic activity the brain has only negligible amounts of energy stores in form of glycogen. Energy reserves are rapidly exhausted and last only for seconds if anaerobic energy production is prevalent (see Mc Ilwain and Bachelard, 1971, for references). The key enzyme in

glycogen mobilization is the glycogen phosphorylase, which is activated by
the allosteric effector 5'AMP. A stimulation by catecholamines, as have
been found for liver and muscle, and the underlying enzyme interconversion
seems also to be present in brain tissue, predominantly in glia cells.

The lack of extensive fuel stores may be necessary. The mammalian brain
is comparatively large, and its metabolic rate is high. To store enough of
the hydrophilic glycogen (fat is not suited as pointed out) the brain would have
to extend in volume with the likely consequence of impaired function.

Vulnerability to Interruption of Energy Production

The mammalian brain is highly aerobic with respect to its metabolism and
extremely vulnerable to disturbances of energy production brought along by
hypoxia, anoxia, ischemia, hypoglycemia etc. This is in part a consequence
of the other features of brain metabolism, but the mechanisms which cause
damage to the brain are not fully understood and the subject of controversy
(Plum, 1973; Hossmann and Kleihues, 1973; Brierley, Meldrum, and Brown,
1973; Cohen, 1973; Symon, 1978)

METABOLIC FEATURES OF BRAINS FROM NONMAMMALIAN ANIMALS

The energy metabolism of the mammalian brain has attracted many students and
has been extensively studied and is therefore fairly well understood. This is
by no means true for the brains of lower vertebrates or even for species
belonging to other phyla. One reason for this may be that there is no direct
medical relevance, another that the brains are much smaller (especially in
relation to the body mass) and not readily available in sufficient amount for
normal biochemical purposes. For that reason indirect methods are often
used. One of these methods, applicable to brains of all sizes, is to determine
the catalytic capacities of enzymes which are representative for important
metabolic pathways. Naturally there exists no direct quantitative correlation
between enzyme activities as measured in vitro under optimal conditions and
the real in vivo events. But if enzyme patterns of different organs or brains
are compared, valuable clues to the metabolic organization, important pathways,
and preponderant fuels can be derived. The enzymatic equipment of an organ
is as characteristic as morphological or structural features are, and it is
the cause of specialization and distinct function. Information gained in this
way can stimulate further studies with more distinct aims.
Another more direct approach, also suitable for many tissues, is to determine
the O_2-consumption and the CO_2-evolution of nervous systems. This method
gives a quantitative account of the energy demand, and using the respiratory
quotient (RQ), an indication of the utilized fuels.

Metabolic Activity and CNS Function

All brains tested so far show a certain level of continuous and spontaneous activity. Additional neuronal function seems to be inseparably connected with energy metabolism exceeding the resting level. Regulation of energy production on the tissue level by regional variations in blood flow and glucose uptake seems to be a phylogenetically old mechanism and is presumably a feature of all vertebrates, since these phenomena could be demonstrated to occur in fish brains (Altenau and Agranoff, 1979). Increased O_2-consumption after electrical stimulation was shown much earlier with isolated CNS of fish and frogs (see Winterstein, 1929). Recently, sophisticated measurements using O_2-microelectrodes showed a local decrease in oxygen tension in activated areas of the tectum opticum in bullfrogs after adequate visual stimulation (Sick and Kreisman, 1979). Brief electrical stimuli produce a transient oxidation of the respiratory chain components in amphibian brains (Moffet and Jöbsis, 1976; Moffet and La Manna, 1978) like those demonstrated in mammals (Rosenthal and Jöbsis, 1971). An increased incorporation of ^{3}H-glucose into the contralateral tectum opticum of monocular frogs after visual stimulation could be detected by means of autoradiography by Wegener (1970). The label was mainly concentrated in the fiber layers where the synapses of the optic nerve terminals are located. In the compound eyes of insects (which in a strict sense do not belong to the CNS) a striking increase of carbohydrate oxidation as well as O_2-consumption was found after illumination (Langer, 1962; Hamdorf and Kaschef, 1964).

Fuels for Energy Production

For all brains tested so far glucose is an adequate fuel. The glycolytic pathway is present and its catalytic capacity is high (see figures 1, 2, and table 1). As in mammals PFK and hexokinase have been identified as regulatory enzymes (Wegener, 1975; Newsholme, Sugden, and Williams, 1977; Strang, Clement, and Rae, 1979). PFK is activated by 5' AMP, K^+, NH_4^+ and inhibited by ATP and, in many cases, by citrate. The effect of citrate can easily be overlooked, since it is abolished at high Mg^{++}-concentration especially with the enzyme from insects (A. Diehl and Wegener, 1980). The exergonic hexokinase reaction is not at the equilibrium (K = [G-6-P] $\cdot$ [ADP] / [Gluc] $\cdot$ [ATP] $\simeq$ 400; Barman, 1969) in brain tissue from all sources as can be seen from the concentrations of glucose and glucose-6-phosphate (table 2). The reversible binding of the enzyme to the mitochondrial membrane seems to be a characteristic of all vertebrate brains, but could not be detected in brain tissue from invertebrate animals (Wegener and Pfeifer, 1975). The contribution of the pentose cycle to the catabolism of glucose seems unimportant with respect to energy production, considering the enzyme activity ratios GAPDH/G6PDH (table 1).

The ability to derive energy anaerobically by production of lactic acid (high LDH activity) is common to most nervous systems. In the brains of cephalopods, however, the capacity is low (Storey, 1977) and it is virtually lacking in the cerebral ganglia of some insects (see fig. 1, 2, and table 1).

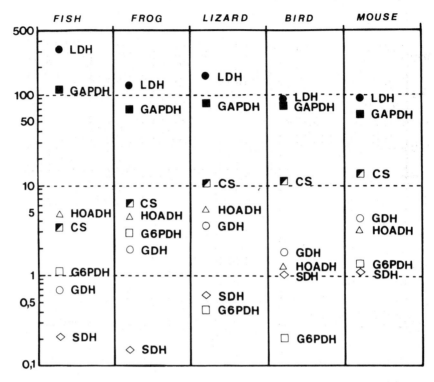

Fig. 1   Metabolic organization in the brains of 5 species
(see table 1), which represent different classes of vertebrates.
Activities (in U/g tissue at 25°C) of enzymes representative for
the main pathways of energy metabolism are given. The catalytic
capacities indicate that carbohydrate is the preponderant fuel and
glycolysis the main pathway in brains from all vertebrates. In
higher classes there is a tendency to increase the capacity of
aerobic oxidations (Data from Wegener and Zebe, 1971).
GAPDH (EC 1.2.1.12): glycolysis; LDH (1.1.1.27): lactate
formation; G-6-PDH (1.1.1.49): pentose cycle; GDH (1.1.1.8):
glycerophosphate cycle; CS (4.1.3.7) and SDH (1.3.99.1):
Krebs cycle; HOADH (1.1.1.35): fatty acid oxidation.

Brains of cephalopods can utilize octopine, a special end product of glycolysis
in molluscs, which is formed instead of lactate by a reductive NADH-dependent
condensation of arginine and pyruvate under anaerobic conditions in some
tissues (muscle e.g.) of these animals. Like lactate this substance can be
delivered to the blood and oxidized by aerobic organs, which in analogy to
the LDH-system have special isoenzymes of the octopine dehydrogenase
(Fields and coworkers, 1976; Storey, 1977; Storey and Storey, 1979a, b).

The ready incorporation of glucose-C into amino acids also seems to be a
common feature for mature nervous tissue, as demonstrated in birds (Lehr
and Gayet, 1976; Lehr, 1979), lower vertebrates (Shank and Baxter, 1973),
as well as in members of other phyla (Bradford and coworkers, 1969).
The capacity to oxidize ketone bodies is common to all brains of vertebrates

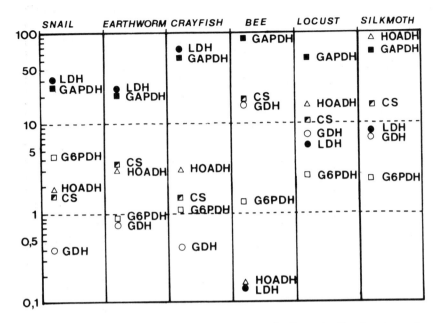

Fig. 2   Organization of energy metabolism in the brains of
6 animals (species see table 1), which represent 3 different phyla.
Insects differ from other forms, they highly depend on
aerobic processes, but have only a low capacity to derive
energy anaerobically by formation of lactic acid. Furthermore some of them like the silkmoth have a high potency
to oxidize fatty acids (Data from Wegener and Zebe, 1973,
and unpublished work).

and invertebrates, since the participating enzymes could be found in all species
tested (Sugden and Newsholme, 1973; B. Diehl and Wegener, unpublished
results).
Another feature, common to all vertebrate brains, is the inability to derive
energy by oxidation of fatty acids. As in mammals, the enzymatic activity
proves to be the limiting factor, since the substrate has easy access to the
cells as demonstrated in the case of fish by Rahmann (1970). Representatives
of other phyla, too, have neglegible capacities to oxidize fatty acids in their
brains compared to other energy yielding pathways (see fig. 2 and table 1).
But the insects again provide remarkable exceptions to this rule. Within this
one class of insects there are species, virtually unable to derive energy from
fat (honey bee, Hymenoptera; blowfly, Diptera), while others, like the silkmoth and some related moths (Lepidoptera) or the locusts (Orthoptera), have
high enzymatic capacity to do so (Wegener and Zebe, 1973; Wegener and
Pfeifer, 1975). This enzymatic capacity is supposed to be used in vivo, since
isolated cerebral ganglia of silkmoths can respire without added substrate at
a high and constant rate (see fig. 3) with an RQ between 0, 7 and 0, 8 (Wegener,
1975). The oxygen consumption is not increased when glucose is added, but
the RQ then seems to be slightly elevated (Wegener, unpublished). These

Table 1   Enzyme activity ratios as indicators of metabolic organization
          in brain tissue from animals, which represent different systematic
          groups.
          GAPDH: glycolysis; LDH: anaerobic glycolysis; G-6-PDH: pentose
          cycle; CS: Krebs cycle; HOADH: FA-oxidation

	$\dfrac{\text{GAPDH}}{\text{LDH}}$	$\dfrac{\text{GAPDH}}{\text{G6PDH}}$	$\dfrac{\text{GAPDH}}{\text{CS}}$	$\dfrac{\text{GAPDH}}{\text{HOADH}}$
Mouse (Mus musculus)	0,6	52,4	4,8	23,7
Bird (Euplectes orix)	0,9	388,0	6,7	63,7
Lizard (Lacerta agilis)	0,5	205,4	7,4	15,6
Frog (Rana esculenta)	0,5	23,1	11,1	15,1
Fish (Carassius c.)	0,3	105,3	36,8	25,5
Silkmoth (Bombyx mori)	6,7	24,3	2,8	0,7
Locust (Locusta migratoria)	9,3	21,1	4,7	3,1
Honey bee (Apis mellifica)	223,3	68,7	4,7	203,0
Crayfish (Orconectes limosus)	0,8	44,4	37,7	17,0
Earthworm (Lumbricus terrestris)	0,9	24,8	6,2	7,1
Snail (Helix pomatia)	0,8	5,9	18,1	14,3

results strongly favor the assumption that a significant amount of energy
is derived from fatty acids, which seem to be an adequate substrate in these
brains. Indeed, fat droplets (triglyceride) could be demonstrated in the CNS
of insects (Wigglesworth, 1960), but never were suspected to be a fuel for
the nervous tissue. This unusual metabolic equipment is supposed to be a
special adaptation to the living conditions of these animals; lepidoptera rely
on fat as the only fuel for flight (Zebe, 1954) and some of them (the silkmoth,
e. g.) never feed as adults.
The catalytic capacity to oxidize fatty acids is acquired during the pupal phase
in the holometabolic forms (Knollmann and Wegener, 1978). At the cell level,
the metabolic differences are a consequence of different specialized mitochondria
present in the tissue. The subcellular metabolic compartmentation proved
to be the same as in mammals (Wegener and Pfeifer, 1975).

Energy Stores

In contrast to mammals, lower vertebrates and the invertebrates tested so
far have significant fuel stores in form of glycogen. Some invertebrate
animals have large amounts of glycogen in their CNS, ranging between
1 and 2 % of the tissue weight (Schallek, 1949; Treherne, 1966). This seems
to be an advantage for many forms in which the circulatory system is not
well developed (open systems in molluscs, arthropods) or substrate homeostasis

Table 2   Glycogen, Glucose, and Glucose-6-Phosphate in the brains or
         other parts of the CNS from different animals in μmole per g
         of tissue

	Glycogen (as Hexose)	Glucose	Glucose-6-P
Mouse (Mus musculus)[1]	2, 2	1, 5	0, 08
Turtle (Pseudemys scripta)[2]	18, 1	2, 0	0, 1
Frog (Rana pipiens)[2]	19, 3	0, 5	0, 1
Fish (Carassius auratus)[2]	12, 8	0, 9	0, 2
Lamprey (Petromyzon marinus)[3]	45, 0	1, 2	0, 1
Locust (Locusta migratoria)[4]	6, 6	1, 0	0, 1
Locust (Schistocerca gregaria)[5] (Thoracic ganglion)	11, 1	1, 7	
Cockroach (Periplaneta americana)[6] (nerve cord)	55, 0		
Spider crab (Libinia emarginata)[7] (CNS-ganglia)	80, 0		

can not readily be maintained, since it provides the nervous system with a
certain degree of metabolic autarchy.
The significance of fuel stores in lower vertebrates is demonstrated by old
observations; the isolated nerve cords of frogs can survive in an oxygen
atmosphere for a day or more (see Winterstein, 1929), isolated frog brains
yield normal EEGs without added substrate for several hours (Libet and
Gerard, 1939).
In the insect nervous system the fuel stores are obviously deposited at
strategically important points. Glycogen was found in the perineurium
enveloping the ganglia, in the glial processes investing the axons, and in the
nerve cells themselves, particularly in the region of the axon cone
(Wigglesworth, 1960; Smith and Treherne, 1963). In the brains of lower
vertebrates glycogen is predominant in the fiber areas and ependymal layers
after application of labelled glucose (Erdmann and Rahmann, 1970; Wegener,
1970). Phosphorylase, the enzyme which breaks down glycogen seems to be
present in all nervous systems. In the frog brain it has features not known from
the corresponding mammalian enzymes.(Kamp and Wegener, 1979). In the
nerve cord of the cockroach the enzyme was shown to be activated by hormonal
factors (Hart and Steele, 1973).

[1] Lowry and coworkers, 1964
[2] Mc Dougal and coworkers, 1968
[3] Rovainen, Lowry, and Passonneau, 1969
[4] Diehl, A., and Wegener, unpublished
[5] Clement and Strang, 1978
[6] Hart and Steele, 1973
[7] Schallek, 1949

Oxygen Consumption and Tolerance to Hypoxia

Brain function depends on aerobic metabolism. In all species tested so far
the CNS is always among the organs with the highest oxygen consumption.
Nevertheless striking differences do exist with respect to the quantitative
aspects of metabolism and to the resistance of the CNS to disturbances in
energy production.
Metabolism is much slower in the brains of lower vertebrates compared to
mammals. Estimates of metabolic rates at 23-25° C in fish, frogs, and
toads, derived from post mortem changes and tracer studies, are between
one-tenth and one-twentieth of the rate in the mouse brain (Mc Dougal and
coworkers, 1968; Shank and Baxter, 1973). In turtle brain even lower values
have been measured. The O_2-consumption of isolated parts of the CNS, too,
is smaller in lower vertebrates (see table 3, where some selected data for
different species are given, for further information see Winterstein, 1929;
Dittmer and Grebe, 1958). This is in accordance with the tendency to increased capacity of aerobic pathways in the brains of animals representing
higher classes of vertebrates (see figure 1 and table 1).
In general, the rate of O_2-uptake of a brain depends on several factors in
a very complex manner, which is not understood in terms of causal relationships. These factors seem to include the body size of the animal, the
efficiency of the CNS, which often reflects the mobility and activity of the
species, and other aspects of living conditions as well as anatomical facts
like the organization of O_2- and substrate-delivering systems.

In most species it is not possible to measure the respiration of the intact
brain in situ. The oxygen uptake of isolated parts of the CNS of course
only can give a rough estimate of the respiratory rate of the tissue in vivo.
Influences of artificial media, the lack of sensory input and neuronal output,
disruption of tissue structure etc. certainly lead to deviations from the
physiological values. In many cases, however, in which the metabolic rates
were determined by different methods or balance-sheets were done, it
could be demonstrated, that in vitro rates are similar or parallel to those
in vivo, thus allowing to estimate the respiratory potential of the organs.
For references see Krebs, 1950; Kerkut and Laverack, 1957; Urich, 1964;
Kleiber, 1965.
Tissue respiration of the highly evolved brain of the active and mobile
cephalopods is fairly high compared to the phylogenetically related but
sluggish snails (table 3). Similar results have been derived by Vernberg
and Gray (1953) and Vernberg (1954) comparing marine teleosts of different
activity levels.

The insects, again, are a special case, their isolated brains, so far tested,
consume 5 ml oxygen or more per gram of wet tissue and hour at 25 ° C
(see table 3 and fig. 3) yielding the highest respiratory rates of brain tissue
ever measured. The high O_2-consumption was also noted by Clement and
Strang (1978) studying the thoracic ganglia of the locust (table 3). These
authors determined the temperature coefficient Q_{10} to be 3,03 between
25° and 35° C.
The higher O_2-uptake measured in our experiments may be due to tissue
differences as well as to different methods. Clement and Strang immersed

Table 3   Oxygen consumption rates (in ml per gram tissue and hour) and respiratory quotients of the human brain and of parts of the CNS from various animals representing different systematic groups

	Conditions	ml O_2/g·h	RQ
Man[1] whole brain	resting adults	2,0	1
Rat[2] whole brain	Animals lightly anesthetized	4,5	1
Frog[3] (Rana temporaria) spinal cord	isolated organ 100 % O_2, 16-18° C	0,23	
Fish[4] (Stenotomus chrysops) brain	tissue homogenate in phosphate buffer, pH 7,5 20 % O_2, 30° C	0,63	
Blowfly[5] (Calliphora erythrocephala) cerebral ganglion	isolated ganglion moistened by saline 20 % O_2, 25° C	7,1	1
Silkmoth[5] (Bombyx mori) cerebral ganglion	isolated ganglion moistened by saline 20 % O_2, 25° C	5,9	0,7-0,8
Locust[6] (Schistocerca gregaria) thoracic ganglia	isolated ganglion in glucose saline 100 % O_2, 35° C 100 % O_2, 25° C	6,8 2,2	
Earthworm[7] (Lumbricus terrestris) nerve cord	isolated nerve cord in buffered saline, pH 7,4 20 % O_2, 25° C	0,33	
Octopus[8] (Eledone cirrhosa) optic lobe	tissue slice in buffered medium plus substrate, pH 7,4, 20 % O_2, 25° C	0,8	
Snail[9] (Helix pomatia) cerebral ganglion	isolated ganglion in Baldwin phosphate, pH 7,4 20 % O_2, 28° C	0,25	

[1] Mc Ilwain and Bachelard, 1971
[2] Nilsson and Siesjö, 1976
[3] Winterstein, 1929
[4] Vernberg, 1954
[5] Wegener, 1975, and unpublished results
[6] Clement and Strang, 1978
[7] Urich, 1964
[8] Bradford and coworkers, 1969; value corrected in accordance with the authors
[9] Kerkut and Laverack, 1957

the isolated ganglia in a fluid medium, while in our studies the brains
were only slightly moistened, in order to keep in function the efficient
O_2-delivering tracheae, which invade the tissues of insects.
It should be mentioned, that the high oxygen uptake is not a special feature
of the nervous system, but is shared with other organs of the insect body.
The brain of a female blowfly e. g. , which is about 0, 8 % of the body mass,
takes up (as an isolated organ) between 3 and 4 % of the total O_2 consumed
by the animal at rest (Kern, Backes, and Wegener, unpublished). The
corresponding figures for man are 2 % and 20-25 % resp. (Mc Ilwain and
Bachelard, 1971).

The pronounced aerobic organization of metabolism in insect brains is a
feature restricted to the adults. It is aquired during the pupal phase in
holometabolic forms (Bernd and Wegener, 1978; Knollmann and Wegener,
1978). In the hemimetabolic locust a decrease of LDH activity is seen around
the nymphal-adult moult (Zimmermann and Wegener, unpublished results).

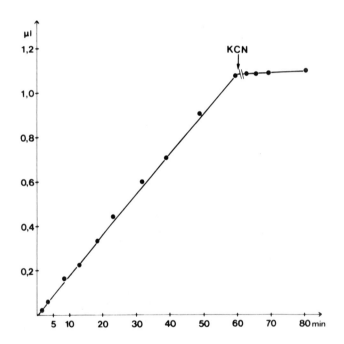

Fig.   3   Oxygen-consumption of the isolated cerebral ganglion
of the silkmoth (Bombyx mori).
The isolated organ was   mounted on a small filter paper,
moistened by 1 µl saline and put into a Hamdorf microrespirometer (Hamdorf and Kaschef, 1964). O_2-uptake is linear for
more than 1 hour without added substrate, it is stopped by
Cyanide.

The extreme vulnerability of the mammalian brain to an interruption of
energy production by hypoxia is well known. The vast majority of animals,
however, are far more tolerant to conditions which rapidly kill mammals.
Adaptations in mammals to hypoxic periods like prolonged diving generally
are believed not to include the brain, but to be a matter of circulatory
changes like bradycardia and extensive peripheral vasoconstriction to
conserve oxygen for the vital organs brain and heart (Andersen, 1966;
Blix and coworkers, 1976). Seals of different species can dive from at
least 15 min up to more than 1 hour, and are outdone by whales (Kooyman,
1972). The above mentioned mechanisms to cope with lack of oxygen are
phylogenetically old and could be demonstrated in many airbreathing
vertebrates and even in fish (Johansen, 1964; Gaunt and Gans, 1969; Smith,
Allison, and Crowder, 1974; Jones and coworkers, 1979).

The resistance to anoxia in several species of lower vertebrates is legendary.
Fish are reported to survive in hermetically sealed glass vessels at $30^{\circ}C$
without food for weeks, reducing their body mass drastically (Mathur, 1967;
see also Coulter, 1967). But the tolerance seems to depend on the species
and the circumstances, like temperature, adaptation etc. Frogs of different
species can easily survive an N_2-atmosphere for more than 1 hour at
room temperature, but the anaerobic energy production cannot maintain
the function of the CNS during the whole time (Mc Dougal and coworkers,
1968; Huhn, Kamp, and Wegener, 1980). The isolated heads of decapitated
turtles show reflex movements for more than 2 hours (Mc Dougal and co-
workers, 1968). The tolerance to anoxia in turtles was shown to correlate
with the buffer capacity (bicarbonate) of the blood (Belkin, 1963), which
is highest in the best divers (8-30 h anoxia, for a review see also Bennett
and Dawson, 1976). These observations point to possibly disastrous effects
of tissue acidosis caused by lactic acid which, for many years, has been
suspected to cause severe effects in mammals (Lindenberg, 1963).
During anoxic conditions the vertebrates rely on glycolysis and formation
of lactic acid as the only important pathway to derive energy from. There
have been suggestions that additional steps can contribute to the energy
metabolism under these conditions. Blazka (1958) reported the anaerobic
accumulation of fatty acids in the carp, but this could not be confirmed by
others (Burton and Spehar, 1971; Driedzic and Hochachka, 1975). The anaerobic production of alanine and of succinate, which theoretically can
yield additional ATP without oxygen, was reported to occur during prolonged
diving periods in mammals and reptiles (Penney, 1974; Hochachka and co-
workers, 1975). The amount of these products, however, is too small to
be significant, and the proposed reactions presumably do not occur in the
CNS. In the rat brain succinate remains at a constant level during hypoxia
(Norberg and Siesjö, 1975b), alanine is only slightly increased (Duffy,
Nelson, and Lowry, 1972; Norberg and Siesjö, 1975b).

Generally the tolerance to hypoxia of the CNS is high, if extensive fuel stores
and sufficient catalytic capacities are available, and in addition, the
metabolic rate is low. This also holds true for the representatives of the
invertebrate phyla, which can roughly be divided into two groups with
respect to their reaction to hypoxia. On the one hand we have species well
adapted to endure long anoxic periods (up to several weeks) without loss of

function, on the other hand we find highly active animals like cephalopods and insects which rapidly loose the ability to react and get paralysed, since their anaerobic energy production is completely insufficient to maintain the CNS function. But anoxic periods often do not cause irreversible damage to the brains in these invertebrates as can be judged from the impressive survival times reported in the literature (for details see the thorough reviews of von Brand, 1934, 1946). Surprisingly the highly active honey bees with their minimal capacity to form lactic acid are reported to survive a severe disturbance of their energy production caused by 100 % CO_2 for 6 hours without changes in behaviour or loss of memory (Medugorac and Lindauer, 1967). Houseflies are immobilised within one minute in an atmosphere of pure nitrogen (Heslop, Price, and Ray, 1963), but nearly all of them recover after 12 hours of anoxia, some even after 24 hours (Engels, 1968a). The maximal survival time depends on the physiological state, the sex and the age of the animals (Engels, 1968b). Using whole flies, Heslop, Price, and Ray (1963) have shown that the concentrations of the "highenergy" compounds ATP and arginine phosphate fall to very low levels within 30 minutes of anaerobiosis, while glycerol 1-phosphate, a typical end product of the anaerobic glycolysis in insects, and inorganic phosphate rise. The metabolic effects of anoxia on the nervous system, however, have not yet been studied in these animals.

Some of the examples given above render it improbable, that it is only the failure of energy that causes neuronal dysfunction and brain damage during hypoxia in mammals. Determinations of the energy status lead to the same conclusion, since neuronal function in mammals fails before the cellular ATP-content decreases signigicantly (see Berntman and Siesjö, 1978a, 1978b, for references).

At the moment we have no reason to postulate adaptions in cell metabolism exceeding mere glycolysis in the brain tissue of vertebrates. Among the species of the many invertebrate phyla, however, which include the vast majority of all living animals special metabolic steps yielding additional ATP can be expected. Recent studies have revealed a variety of biochemical adaptations to life without oxygen including the production of ethanol, polyols, glycerol, alanine, succinate, and volatile fatty acids (von Brand, 1973; Hochachka, Fields, and Mustafa, 1973; Grieshaber and Gäde, 1976; Schöttler and Schroff, 1976; Zebe, 1977).

These studies, however, do not refer to nervous tissue (the few exceptions are mentioned above), but are performed with whole animals or muscle tissue. Further research must clarify whether reactions exceeding glycolysis are significant for the anaerobic energy production in nervous systems. It is of considerable interest in this context, that the invertebrate groups with the highest tolerance of anoxia do not accumulate lactic acid during anaerobiosis.

From our comparative considerations it seems likely that the vulnerability of the mammalian brain is the price to be paid for the high efficiency of that organ, which is not burdened with large fuel stores but relies on an intricate circulation providing substrates and allowing an efficient aerobic metabolism. These features again are based on the impressive homeostasis of the mammalian body.

OUTLOOK

To guarantee the brains' permanent energy supply and to avoid disturbances caused by events in other parts of the body are central problems for all animals. Structure and function of nerve cells are similar in the whole animal kingdom and the basic aspects of metabolism and subcellular compartmentation in all brains tested so far are similar, too. Nevertheless different adaptations have been developed in different groups to reach the above mentioned aims, enabling animals to live under a variety of living conditions. In most animals the means to ensure a proper functioning of the brain include blood-brain-barrier systems, energy stores, and restriction of certain metabolic capacities in the CNS.

The mammalian brain, as a special case, has no fuel stores, but relies on the impressive caloric homeostasis, resulting in an outstanding CNS-efficiency on one hand but leading to high vulnerability and sensitivity on the other. Therefore the more resistent lower brains often are better suited to answer basic neurobiological problems. Moreover some of the metabolic peculiarities of mammalian brains may be elucidated studying lower animals. For example metabolic events can be followed on an extended time scale in lower vertebrates on the basis of their slower brain metabolism. The consequences of permanent blood supply by capillaries and the critical recirculation after extended hypoxia may be elucidated by comparing to forms which do not have a closed circulatory system. The effects of tissue acidosis can be evaluated by comparison to species which do not produce lactic acid during anaerobiosis. In this way the basic research on lower animals may well contribute to a better understanding of the intricate metabolism of the mammalian brain.

ACKNOWLEDGEMENT

Thanks are due to Mrs. Ingelore Piella for skilful technical assistance and to my students and coworkers for their engaged work.
The measurements on isolated insect ganglia were performed mainly with a microrespirometer provided by Prof. Hamdorf (Bochum). The help by him and by his collaborators, especially Miss Petra Jergolla and Dr. G. Rosner is gratefully acknowledged.
Our work was supported by Deutsche Forschungsgemeinschaft, Bonn-Bad Godesberg.

REFERENCES

Altenau, L. L., and B. W. Agranoff (1979). Visual stimulation increases regional cerebral blood flow and metabolism in the Goldfish. Brain Res., 161, 55-61.

Andersen, H. T. (1966). Physiological adaptations in diving vertebrates. Physiol. Rev., 46, 212-243.

Barman, T. E. (1969). Enzyme Handbook I. Springer, Berlin, New York.

Belkin, D. A. (1963). Anoxia: Tolerance in reptiles. Science, 139, 492-493.

Bennett, A. F., and W. R. Dawson (1976). Metabolism. In C. Gans (Ed.), Biology of the Reptilia, Vol. 5, 127-223. Academic Press, New York.

Bernd, A., and G. Wegener (1978). Änderungen der Stoffwechselorganisation von Insektengehirnen im Verlaufe der Ontogenese: Aktivitätsmuster von Enzymen des Grundstoffwechsels bei der Fliege (Calliphora erythrocephala). Verh. Dtsch. Zool. Ges. 1978, 275. G. Fischer, Stuttgart.

Berntman, L., and B. K. Siesjö (1978a). Cerebral metabolic and circulatory changes induced by hypoxia in starved rats. J. Neurochem., 31, 1265-1276.

Berntman, L., and B. K. Siesjö (1978b). Brain energy metabolism and circulation in hypoxia. In: V. Neuhoff (Ed.), Proc. Europ. Soc. Neurochem., 1, 253-265. Verlag Chemie, Weinheim and New York.

Blazka, P. (1958). The anaerobic metabolism of fish. Physiol. Zool., 31, 117-128.

Blix, A. S., J. K. Kjekshus, I. Enge, and A. Bergan (1976). Myocardial blood flow in the diving seal. Acta Physiol. Scand., 96, 277-280.

Bradford, H. F., E. B. Chain, H. T. Cory, and S. P. R. Rose (1969). Glucose and amino acid metabolism in some invertebrate nervous systems. J. Neurochem., 16, 969-978.

Brand, T. von (1934). Das Leben ohne Sauerstoff bei wirbellosen Tieren. Ergebn. Biol., 10, 37-100.

Brand, T. von (1946). Anaerobiosis in invertebrates. Biodynamica, Normandy 21, Missouri.

Brand, T. von (1973). Biochemistry of Parasites. Academic Press, New York.

Brierley, J. B., B. S. Meldrum, and A. W. Brown (1973). The threshold and neuropathology of cerebral "anoxic-ischemic" cell change. Arch. Neurol. (Chic.), 29, 367-374.

Burton, D. T., and A. M. Spehar (1971). A re-evaluation of the anaerobic end products of fresh-water fish exposed to environmental hypoxia. Comp. Biochem. Physiol., 40A, 945-954.

Cahill, G. F., O. E. Owen, and A. P. Morgan (1968). The consumption of fuels during prolonged starvation. Adv. Enzyme Reg., 6, 143-150.

Clement, E. M., and R. H. C. Strang (1978). A Comparison of some aspects of the physiology and metabolism of the nervous system of the locust Schistocerca gregaria in vitro with those in vivo. J. Neurochem., 31, 135-145.

Cohen, M. M. (Ed.) (1973). Biochemistry, Ultrastructure, and Physiology of Cerebral Anoxia, Hypoxia and Ischemia. Karger, New York.

Coulter, G. W. (1967). Low apparent oxygen requirements of deep water fishes in Lake Tanganyika. Nature (London), 215, 317-318.

Cremer, J. E. (1964). Amino acid metabolism in rat brain studied with ^{14}C-labelled glucose. J. Neurochem. (Oxford), 11, 165-185.

Dhopeshwarkar, G. A., and J. F. Mead (1973). Uptake and transport of fatty acids into the brain and the role of the blood-brain barrier system. Adv. Lipid Res., 11, 109-142.

Diehl, A., and G. Wegener (1980). Die regulatorischen Eigenschaften der 6-Phosphofructokinase aus dem Nervengewebe von Insekten. Hoppe Seyler's Z. Physiol. Chemie, in press.

Dittmer, D. S., and R. M. Grebe (Eds.) (1958). Handbook of Respiration. Saunders Comp., Philadelphia and London.

Driedzic, W. R., and P. W. Hochachka (1975). The unanswered question of high anaerobic capabilities of carp white muscle. Can. J. Zoology, 53, 706-712.

Duffy, T. E., S. R. Nelson, and O. H. Lowry (1972). Cerebral carbo-hydrate metabolism during acute hypoxia and recovery. J. Neurochem., 19, 959-977.

Engels, W. (1968a). Anaerobioseversuche mit Musca domestica. Alters- und Geschlechtsunterschiede von Überlebensrate und Erholfähigkeit. J. Insect Physiol., 14, 253-260.

Engels, W. (1968b). Anaerobioseversuche mit Musca domestica. Ver-wertung normaler und experimentell erzeugter Kohlenhydratreser-ven. J. Insect Physiol., 14, 869-879.

Erdmann, G., and H. Rahmann (1970). Einfluß von Acetoxycycloheximid (Actidion) auf die Protein- und Glykogensynthese im ZNS von Teleosteern. Cytobiologie, 1, 468-481.

Fields, J., H. Guderley, K. B. Storey, P. W. Hochachka (1976). The pyruvate branchpoint in squid brain: Competition between octopine dehydrogenase and lactate dehydrogenase. Can. J. Zoology, 54, 879-885.

Gaitonde, M. K., D. R. Dahl, and K. A. C. Elliot (1965). Entry of glucose carbon into amino acids of rat brain and liver in vivo after injection of uniformly ^{14}C-labelled glucose. Biochem. J., 94, 345-352.

Gaitonde, M. K., S. A. Marchi, and D. Richter (1964). The utilization of glucose in the brain and other organs of the cat. Proc. R. Soc. B., 160, 124-136.

Gaunt, A. S., and C. Gans (1969). Diving bradycardia and withdrawal brady-cardia in Caiman crocodilus. Nature (London), 223, 207-208.

Grieshaber, M., and G. Gäde (1976). The biological role of octopine in the squid Loligo vulgaris. J. Comp. Physiol., 108, 225-232.

Hamdorf, K., and A. H. Kaschef (1964). Der Sauerstoffverbrauch des Facetten-auges von Calliphora erythrocephala in Abhängigkeit von der Temperatur und dem Ionenmilieu. Z. vergl. Physiol., 48, 251-265.

Hart, D. E., and J. E. Steele (1973). The glycogenolytic effect of the corpus cardiacum on the cockroach nerve cord. J. Insect Physiol., 19, 927-939.

Hawkins, R. A., and J. F. Biebuyck (1979). Ketone bodies are selectively used by individual brain regions. Science, 205, 325-327.

Hawkins, R. A., D. H. Williamson, and H. A. Krebs (1971). Ketone body utilization by adult and suckling rat brain in vivo. Biochem. J., 122, 13-18.

Heslop, J. P., G. M. Price, and J. W. Ray (1963). Anaerobic metabolism in the housefly, Musca domestica L. Biochem. J., 87, 35-38.

Hochachka, P., J. Fields, and T. Mustafa (1973). Animal life without oxygen: Basic biochemical mechanisms. American Zoologist, 13, 543-555.

Hochachka, R. W., T. G. Owen, J. F. Allen, and G. C. Whittow (1975).
    Multiple end products of anaerobiosis in diving vertebrates. Comp. Biochem.
    Physiol., 50 B, 17-22.
Hossmann, K. A., and P. Kleihues (1973). Reversibility of ischemic brain
    damage. Archs. Neurol. (Chic.)., 29, 375-384.
Hostetler, K. Y., and B. R. Landau (1967). Estimation of the pentose cycle
    contribution to glucose metabolism in tissue in vivo. Biochemistry (Wash.),
    6, 2961-2964.
Hostetler, K. Y., B. R. Landau, R. J. White, M. S. Albin, and D. Yashon
    (1970). Contribution of the pentose cycle to the metabolism of glucose in
    the isolated perfused brain of the monkey. J. Neurochem., 17, 33-39.
Huhn, H., G. Kamp, and G. Wegener (1980). Der Glykogenstoffwechsel im Ge-
    hirn des Frosches bei normaler, verminderter und erhöhter Sauerstoffzufuhr.
    Verh. Dtsch. Zool. Ges. 1980, in press.
Ingvar, D. H., and N. A. Lassen (Eds.) (1975). Brain work: The coupling of
    function, metabolism and blood flow in the brain. Munksgaard, Copenhagen.
Jöbsis, F. F., M. O`Connor, M. Uitale, and H. Ureman (1971). Intracellular
    redox changes in functioning cerebral cortex. I. Metabolic effects of
    epileptiform activity. J. Neurophysiol., 34, 735-749.
Joel, C. D., C. A. Ellis, J. K. Lace, P. B. Joel, M. R. Swanson, and
    J. R. Stroemer (1974). Stability of the brain fatty acid pattern in adult rats
    during extreme starvation. J. Neurochem., 23, 23-28.
Johansen, K. (1964). Regional distribution of circulating blood during submersion
    asphyxia in the duck. Acta Physiol. Scand., 62, 1-9.
Jones, D. R., R. M. Bryan, jr., N. H. West, R. H. Lord, B. Clark (1979).
    Regional distribution of blood flow during diving in the duck (Anas
    platyrhynchos). Can. J. Zoology, 57, 995-1002.
Kamp, G., and G. Wegener (1979). Properties of glycogen phosphorylase from
    brain tissue of frogs. Abstr. FEBS Meeting on Enzymes 1979, S 1-148.
Kerkut, G. A., and M. S. Laverack (1957). The respiration of Helix pomatia,
    a balance sheet. J. exp. Biol., 34, 97-105.
Kleiber, M. (1965). Respiratory exchange and metabolic rate. In: W. O. Fenn,
    and H. Rahn (Eds.), Handbook of Physiology, Section 3, Vol. II, 927-938.
    American Physiological Society, Washington.
Knollmann, U., and G. Wegener (1978). Zum Energiestoffwechsel in den Gehir-
    nen von Insekten: Enzymaktivitätsmuster der Cerebralganglien von Bombyx
    mori in 3 Stadien der Ontogenese. Verh. Dtsch. Zool. Ges.1978, 292.
    G. Fischer, Stuttgart.
Knull, H. R., W. F. Taylor, and W. W. Wells (1973). Effects of energy
    metabolism on in vivo distribution of hexokinase in brain. J. Biol. Chem.,
    248, 5414-5417.
Kooyman, G. L. (1972). Deep diving behaviour and effects of pressure in reptiles,
    birds, and mammals. Soc. exp. Biol. Symp., 26, 295-311.
Krebs, H. A. (1950). Body size and tissue respiration. Biochim. biophys. Acta
    (Amst.), 4, 249-269.
Langer, H. (1962). Untersuchungen über die Größe des Stoffwechsels isolierter
    Augen von Calliphora erythrocephala Meigen. Biol. Zentralbl., 81, 691-720.
Lassen, N. A., D. H. Ingvar, E. Skinhøj (1978). Brain function and blood flow
    (patterns of activity in the human cerebral cortex are graphically displayed).
    Scientific American, 239 (4), 62-71.
Lehr, P. R. (1979). Utilization in vivo of glucose carbon in the optic lobes and

the cerebellum of the chick during postnatal growth. Comp. Biochem. Physiol.,
    63 B, 267-273.
Lehr, P. R., and J. Gayet (1976). Kinetics of utilization in vivo of glucose
    carbon in the chick cerebral hemispheres during postnatal growth. Comp.
    Biochem. Physiol., 53 B, 215-224.
Libet, B., and R. W. Gerard (1939). Control of the potential rhythm of the isolated
    frog brain. J. Neurophysiol., 2, 153-169.
Lindenberg, R. (1963). Patterns of CNS vulnerability in acute hypoxaemia, in-
    cluding anaesthesia accidents. In: Schadé, J. P., and W. H. Mc Menemey (Eds.),
    Selective vulnerability of the brain in hypoxaemia. Blackwell, Oxford.
Lowry, O. H., J. V. Passonneau, F. X. Hasselberger, and D. W. Schulz (1964).
    Effect of ischemia on known substrates and cofactors of the glycolytic pathway
    in brain. J. biol. Chem., 239, 18-30.
Mathur, G. B. (1967). Anaerobic respiration in a cyprinoid fish Rasbora
    daniconius (Ham). Nature, 214, 318-319.
Mc Dougal, D. B. jr., J. Holowach, M. C. Howe, E. M. Jones, and C. A. Thomas
    (1968). The effects of anoxia upon energy sources and selected metabolic inter-
    mediates in the brains of fish, frog and turtle. J. Neurochem., 15, 577-588.
Mc Ilwain, H., and H. S. Bachelard (1971). Biochemistry and the central nervous
    system. 4th ed. Churchill, London.
Medugorac, I., and M. Lindauer (1967). Das Zeitgedächtnis der Bienen unter dem
    Einfluß von Narkose und von sozialen Zeitgebern. Z. vergl. Physiol., 55, 450-474.
Moffet, D. F., and F. F. Jöbsis (1976). Response of toad brain respiratory chain
    enzymes to ouabain, elevated potassium, and electrical stimulus. Brain
    Research, 117, 239-255.
Moffet, D. F., and J. La Manna (1978). Contributions of glycolysis and oxidative
    metabolism to recovery from electrical pulse in the isolated toad brain. Brain
    Research, 152, 365-368.
Newsholme, E. A., P. H. Sugden, and T. Williams (1977). Effect of citrate on
    the activities of 6-phosphofructokinase from nervous and muscle tissues from
    different animals and its relationship to the regulation of glycolysis. Biochem. J.,
    166, 123-129.
Nilsson, B., and B. K. Siesjö (1976). A method for determining blood flow and
    oxygen consumption in the rat brain. Acta Physiol. Scand., 96, 72-82.
Norberg, K., and B. K. Siesjö (1975 a). Cerebral metabolism in hypoxic hypoxia.
    I. Pattern of activation of glycolysis, a re-evaluation. Brain Research, 86, 31-44.
Norberg, K., and B. K. Siesjö (1975 b). Cerebral metabolism in hypoxic hypoxia.
    II. Citric acid cycle intermediates and associated amino acids. Brain Research,
    86, 45-54.
Norberg, K., and B. K. Siesjö (1976). Oxidative metabolism of the cerebral cortex
    of the rat in severe insulin-induced hypoglycemia. J. Neurochem., 26, 345-352.
Penney, D. G. (1974). Effects of prolonged diving anoxia on the turtle, Pseudemys
    scripta elegans. Comp. Biochem. Physiol., 47 A, 933-941.
Plum, F. (1973). The clinical problem: How much anoxia-ischemia damages the
    brain? Arch. Neurol. (Chic.), 29, 359-360.
Rahmann, H. (1970). Transport von 3H-Palmitinsäure im ZNS von Teleosteern.
    Z. Zellforschung, 110, 444-456.
Raichle, M. E., R. L. Grubb, H. G. Mokhtar, J. O. Eichling, and M. M.
    Terpogossian (1976). Correlation between regional cerebral blood flow and
    oxidative metabolism. Arch. Neurol., 33, 523-526.
Rosenthal, M., and F. F. Jöbsis (1971). Intracellular redox changes in functioning

cerebral cortex. II. Effects of direct cortical stimulation. J. Neurophysiol.,
34, 750-762.

Rovainen, C. M., O. H. Lowry, and J. V. Passonneau (1969). Levels of metabolites
and production of glucose in the lamprey brain. J. Neurochem., 16, 1451-1458.

Schallek, W. (1949). The glycogen content of some invertebrate nerves. Biol. Bull.,
97, 252-253.

Schöttler, U., and G. Schroff (1976). Untersuchungen zum anaeroben Glykogenabbau
bei Tubifex. J. Comp. Physiol., 108, 243-254.

Scow, R. O., and S. S. Chernick (1970). Mobilization, transport and utilization
of free fatty acids. In: Florkin, M., and E. H. Stotz (Eds.), Comprehensive
biochemistry, Vol. 18, Lipid metabolism, 19-49. Elsevier Publ. Comp., New Yor

Shank, R. P., and C. F. Baxter (1973). Metabolism of glucose, amino acids, and
some related metabolites in the brain of toads (Bufo boreas) adapted to fresh
water and hyperosmotic environments. J. Neurochem., 21, 301-313.

Shimada, M., T. Kihara, K. Kurimoto, and M. Watanabe (1973). Incorporation
of ^{14}C from U-^{14}C glucose into free amino acids in mouse brain loci in vivo
under normal conditions. J. Neurochem., 20, 1337-1344.

Sick, T. J., and N. R. Kreisman (1979). Local tissue oxygen tension as an index
of changes in oxidative metabolism in the bullfrog optic tectum. Brain Research,
169, 575-579.

Smith, D. S., and J. E. Treherne (1963). Functional aspects of the organization
of the insect nervous system. In: Beament, J. W. L., J. E. Treherne, and
V. B. Wigglesworth (Eds.), Advances in Insect Physiology, 1, 401-484.

Smith, E. N., R. D. Allison, and W. E. Crowder (1974). Bradycardia in a free-
ranging american alligator. Copeia 1974: 770-772.

Sokoloff, L. (1973). Metabolism of the ketone bodies by the brain. Ann. Rev. Med.,
24, 271-288.

Sokoloff, L. (1977). Relation between physiological function and energy metabolism
in the central nervous system. J. Neurochem., 29, 13-26.

Sokoloff, L., M. Reivich, C. Kennedy, M. H. de Rosiers, C. S. Patlak, K. D.
Pettigrew, O. Sakurada, and M. Shinonara (1977). The ^{14}C deoxyglucose
method for the measurement of local cerebral glucose utilization: theory,
procedure, and normal values in conscious and anesthetized albino rat.
J. Neurochem., 28, 897-916.

Storey, K. B. (1977). Tissue specific isoenzymes of octopine dehydrogenase in the
cuttlefish, Sepia officinalis. The roles of octopine dehydrogenase and lactate
dehydrogenase in Sepia. J. Comp. Physiol., 115, 159-169.

Storey, K. B., and J. M. Storey (1979 a). Octopine metabolism in the cuttlefish,
Sepia officinalis. Octopine production by muscle and its role as an aerobic
substrate for non-muscular tissues. J. Comp. Physiol., 131, 311-319.

Storey, K. B., and J. M. Storey (1979 b). Kinetic characterization of tissue-
specific isoenzymes of octopine dehydrogenase from mantle muscle and brain
of Sepia officinalis. Functional similarities to the M_4 and H_4 isozymes of
lactate dehydrogenase. Eur. J. Biochem., 93, 545-552.

Strang, R. H. C., E. M. Clement, and R. C. Rae (1979). Some aspects of the
carbohydrate metabolism of the thoracic ganglia of the locust, Schistocerca
gregaria. Comp. Biochem. Physiol., 62 B, 217-224.

Sugden, P. H., and E. A. Newsholme (1973). Activities of hexokinase, phosphofructokinase, 3-oxo acid coenzyme A-transferase and acetoacetyl-coenzyme A
thiolase in nervous tissue from vertebrates and invertebrates. Biochem. J.,
134, 97-101.

Symon, L. (1978). Clinical aspects of anoxia in the nervous system. V. Neuhoff
    (Ed.). Proc. Europ. Soc. Neurochem., 1, 239-252. Verlag Chemie, Weinheim.
Treherne, J. E. (1966). The Neurochemistry of Arthropods. Cambridge Monographs
    in Experimental Biology, No. 14. Cambridge University Press, London.
Urich, K. (1964). Die endogene Atmung der isolierten Organe beim Regenwurm
    Lumbricus terrestris L. Z. vergl. Physiol., 48, 190-197.
Vallejo, C. G., R. Marco, and J. Sebastian (1970). The assoziation of brain
    hexokinase with mitochondrial membranes and its functional implications. Eur.
    J. Biochem., 14, 478-485.
Vernberg, F. J. (1954). The respiratory metabolism of tissues of marine teleosts
    in relation to activity and body size. Biol. Bull., 106, 360-370.
Vernberg, F. J., and J. E. Gray (1953). A comparative study of the respiratory
    metabolism of excised brain tissue of marine teleosts. Biol. Bull., 104, 445-449.
Vrba, R. (1962). Glucose metabolism in rat brain in vivo. Nature, 195, 663-665.
Vrba, R., M. K. Gaitonde, and D. Richter (1962). The conversion of glucose
    carbon into protein in the brain and other organs of the rat. J. Neurochem., 9,
    465-475.
Wegener, G. (1970). Autoradiographische Untersuchungen über gesteigerte Protein-
    synthese im Tectum opticum von Fröschen nach optischer Reizung. Diss. Math.
    Nat. Fak. Westf. Wilhelms Univ., 48, 39-40. Aschendorff, Münster.
Wegener, G. (1975). Comparative biochemistry of energy metabolism in brain
    tissue from insects. Abstr. 10th FEBS-Meeting, 1554. Société de Chimie
    Biologique, Paris.
Wegener, G., and J. Pfeifer (1975). Besonderheiten der Stoffwechselorganisation
    in den Hirnen von Vertebraten und Evertebraten. Verh. Dtsch. Zool. Ges. 1974,
    266-271. G. Fischer, Stuttgart.
Wegener, G., and E. Zebe (1971). Zum Energiestoffwechsel des Gehirns. Eine
    vergleichende Untersuchung an Vertretern der verschiedenen Wirbeltierklassen.
    Z. vergl. Physiol., 73, 195-208.
Wegener, G., and E. Zebe (1973). Zum Energiestoffwechsel in den Hirnen wirbel-
    loser Tiere. Naturwissenschaften, 60, 551-552.
Wigglesworth, B. V. (1960). The nutrition of the central nervous system in the
    cockroach Periplaneta americana L. The role of perineuricum and glial cells
    in the mobilization of reserves. Exp. Biol., 37, 500-512.
Wilson, J. E. (1968). Brain hexokinase. A proposed relation between soluble -
    particulate distribution and activity in vivo. J. Biol. Chem., 243, 3640-3647.
Winterstein, H. (1929). Der Stoffwechsel des Zentralnervensystems. In: Bethe, A.,
    G. v. Bergmann, G. Emben, and A. Ellinger (Eds.), Handbuch der normalen
    und pathologischen Physiologie. Band 9, 515-611. Springer, Berlin.
Zebe, E. (1954). Über den Stoffwechsel der Lepidopteren. Z. vergl. Physiol.,
    36, 290-317.
Zebe, E. (1977). Anaerober Stoffwechsel bei wirbellosen Tieren. Rhein. Westf.
    Akad. Wissensch., N 269, 51-73. Westdeutscher Verlag.

DISCUSSION

<u>Sokoloff</u>:   Thank you Dr. Wegener for this fascinating lecture on comparative biochemistry. Do insects have CO_2 fixing enzymes? Did you look on this?

<u>Wegener</u>:   They have, but nothing is known on these enzymes from brain tissue. We have no yet studied this topic, but CO_2-fixation in the tissue certainly can not account for the low RQ of the brains in some insects.

<u>Hoyer</u>:   One short comment: We measured brain blood flow and metabolism in dementia patients and we found in the initial phase a normal cerebral blood flow and a normal CMR oxygen but the CMR glucose was decreased as well as the respiratory quotient was. And we found a positive cerebral A-V difference of short chained fatty acids. Our assumption was that these fatty acids were burnt in the brains of these patients instead of glucose. Would it be possible that men would have enzymes to use fatty acids or are these fatty acids taken up as a sign of a pathological process?

<u>Wegener</u>:   I suppose, that the oxidation of ketone bodies could cause the lowered RQ.

<u>Hoyer</u>:   Ketone bodies might be used by the brain but only in case of starvation. But these patients did not starve.

<u>Wegener</u>:   And they had no ketone bodies?

<u>Hoyer</u>:   They had, of course, but at normal levels. There was no A-V difference of the brain under these conditions. The A-V difference was zero. But there was an uptake of short chained fatty acids.

<u>Wegener</u>:   A slight enzymatic activity of the fatty acids degrading enzymes is found in the brain, but this is negligible with respect to energy production. Even in ruminants, which get most of their energy from the metabolism of volatile fatty acids, these play no significant role for the brain.

<u>Sokoloff</u>:   Cahill's group studied ketone bodies in starving human subjects and were the first to report the actual utilization of ketone by brain in starvation. They looked at the arteriovenous fatty acid differences, and they were negliible. Normal brain in starving patients has very little capability of utilizing fatty acids.

<u>Hoyer</u>:   That's right. That's normal in normal patients, but not in dementia patients. I think that it is different as it is in amino acids. The A-V difference in normals is zero, but in dementia patients, the A-V difference can be very high.

<u>Andjus</u>:   Is there any possibility in your opinion, including limbic brain,to use fatty acids under strictly anaerobic conditions as a source of energy?

<u>Wegener</u>:   These mechanisms are not knwon from insects, nor from any other group of animals. The larvae of insects, however, do have different mechanisms to cope with anoxia; and adult insects in spite of their highly active CNS-metabolism can survive extended periods of anoxia without damage, as J. P. Heslop demonstrated

some 15 years ago. But I think fatty acids are not involved.

Andjus: So do I. But many people think that there is a fatty acids metabolism under anaerobic conditions.

Wegener: I do not think so and earlier reports on lower vertebrates concerning this topic could not be confirmed later.

Andjus: So they can not make use of that possibility of the stores in the brain of the fatty acids unter anaerobic conditions.

Wegener: Yes, I agree.

Porsche: In some special metabolic situations, e.g. perinatal time or prolonged starvation in animals, the enzymatic pattern of some organs, e.g. liver and kidney, changes. The main substrate for the energy supply instead of glucose are the triglycerids; also glucose, in small amounts, resulting from gluconeogenesis will be utilized. Enhanced resistance of the newborn to hypoxia and anoxia was observed, too. It is possible that the pathological changes of the metabolism in senile dementia induce changes of enzymatic activities associated with an increase in utilization of fatty acids in the brain.

Wegener: The enzyme pattern of the adult mammalian brain is fairly constant. During the perinatal phase, however, the activities of ketone body oxidizing enzymes change markedly, no comparable changes in fatty acid oxidizing enzymes are known. To my knowledge mammalian brains can not derive energy from fatty acid under physiological conditions, and in senile dementia perhaps ketone bodies are involved too.

Hoyer: Another point is whether the human brain is capable to use fatty acids. Is this capacity only present at the perinatal phase and decreases after this period since the oxidative and the glycolytic processes will take part more and more in the metabolism.

Sokoloff: But you can't get energy from fatty acids.

Hoyer: Then they are taken up but not used.

Sokoloff: They are may be incorporated in triglycerides and fat.

Anoxic Rat Model

V. Stefanovich

Hoechst Aktiengesellschaft, Frankfurt am Main, Werk Albert,
6200 Wiesbaden 12, Federal Republic of Germany

ABSTRACT

An anoxic rat model is described in which Sprague-Dawley rats are breathing nitrogen for 30 s. This short period of anoxia is producing a deep disturbance in the
energy metabolism and in the cyclic nucleotide metabolism in rat brain.
It is suggested that this model can be used in the search for a new pharmacological agent able to reverse the metabolic changes caused by anoxia.

KEYWORDS

Anoxic rat model; 30 s N_2 breathing; 10 % O_2 hypoxia; cerebral energy metabolism.

INTRODUCTION

It is well established by Siesjö (1977) that hypoxia has only when sufficiently severe or sufficiently long, a profound influence on the brain energy production -
at the end it leads also to irreversible neuronal damage. Before this end stage is
reached however, compensatory mechanisms are initiated involving change in the
cerebral blood flow (CBF) and in cerebral metabolism.
In view of only minor changes in the metabolism caused by an incomplete hypoxia or
hypoxia of a short duration, it was of interest to study changes in cerebral metabolism in the rat exposed to pure nitrogen breathing for 30 s. This short period
of anoxia caused the dramatic changes in the metabolism of rat brain, summarized
in this report.

MATERIALS AND METHODS

In all experiments Sprague-Dawley rats (females, weight 200 - 220 grs) were used.
Rats were fed Altromin[R] 1314 and water ad libitum. In experiments where rats
were exposed to the atmosphere of 10 % of oxygen, the hypoxy chamber was used
(Fig. 1).

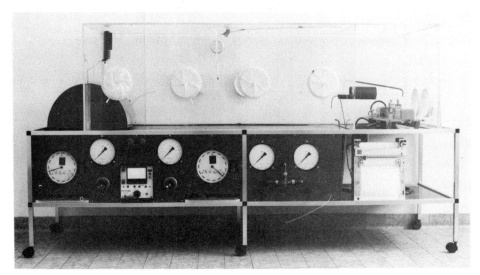

Fig. 1. The hypoxy chamber constructed in the Dept. of
Biochemistry, Hoechst AG, Werk Albert, by
Mr. Gojowczyk.

This chamber had a total volume of 760 l (pre-chamber with a brain-blower has a volume of 110 l) and a gas mixture flow was 625 - 650 l per hr. At the end of the experiment, animals were sacrified by a brain-blower as described by Veech and others (1973).

In experiments with anoxic rats, Sprague-Dawley rats were positioned in the brain-blower and were subjected to breathing pure nitrogen for 30 s. This was done by passing a stream of nitrogen through rubber tubing (∅ 7 mm) at the distance of 10 mm from the rat nose. The rate of the nitrogen flow was 15 l/min. After 30 s rats were sacrified by the brain freezing method using modified Veech's brain-blower shown on the Fig. 2.

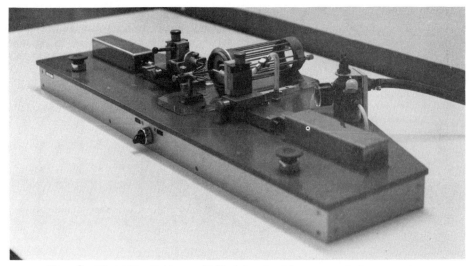

Fig. 2. Picture of the modified brain-blower used for sacri-
fice of rats.

The apparatus was modified in such a way that the moving parts with the hollow probes are activated by air-pressure and not as originally constructed with electro magnets. The hollow probes are forced into the scull and the supratentorial parts of the brain are blown out and frozen to a thin layer in an aluminium chamber at liquid nitrogen temperature.
Before being sacrificed, the experimental rats breathed pure nitrogen for 30 s. The control rats breathed air. After removal, the brain tissue was ground to a powder under liquid nitrogen and extracted as described by McMillan and Siesjö (1972). Fluorimetric, enzymatic determination of cerebral metabolites was performed according to McMillan and Siesjö (1972) or according to Bergmeyer (1974).
The adenylate energy charge (AEC) was calculated according to Atkinson (1968). In experiments with a recovery period, rats, after 30 s of nitrogen breathing, spontaneously breathed air for 5 min. After that time, rats were sacrificed by brainblower and brain metabolites determined as described.
The determination of the body temperature was accomplished by vaginal insertion of an electronic thermometer and recording of the temperature.

Arterial oxygen tension (P_a O_2), carbon dioxide (P_a CO_2), as well as pH, were determined in the following manner. Rats were briefly anesthetized with halothane and situated in a specially constructed restraining cage. Femoral artery and femoral vein were cannulated for blood withdrawal. 20 min later P_a O_2, P_a CO_2 and pH were measured in normal blood by a blood gas analyser Radiometer (Copenhagen) model BMS 3 Mk 2 Blood micro system.
After 30 s of nitrogen breathing arterial blood sample was withdrawn again and P_a O_2, P_a CO_2 and pH measured.

For the determination of cardiovascular parameters rats were briefly anesthetized with halothane and situated in a special restraining cage. The femoral artery and the femoral vein were isolated and cannulated. Recording (Brush recorder, model 481) has started after 20 min of a steady state period. During the following minutes normal values were obtained. Measurements were continued during 30 s when rat was breathing nitrogen and 10 s later during the recovery period (air breathing). In experiments where cyclic nucleotide systems in rat brain were examined, normal rats and rats after breathing nitrogen for 30 s were sacrificed by the brainblower.

Adenylate cyclase and guanylate cyclase were determined by conversion of the nucleotide phosphates into the corresponding cyclic nucleotides. The later were measured by a radio and radioimmune assays respectively using Amersham test kits. The total procedure was similar to one described by Shier and others (1976).

cAMP and cGMP phosphodiesterases (cAMP PDE and cGMP PDE) were determined in rats brain by the method of Pichard and Cheung (1976).
Protein was determined by the method of Gornall and others (1949).

        RESULTS

The results of the determination of some of the cerebral metabolites in the brain of the rats subjected to hypoxia (10 % O_2 for a week) and control rats, are shown in Table 1.

V. Stefanovich

TABLE 1   Influence of Hypoxia (one week at 10 % O$_2$) on Adenine
nucleotides, Lactate and Pyruvate content of Rat Brain

Metabolite μmol/g wet tissue	Normoxia	Hypoxia	Change in %
ATP	2.794 + 0.138	2.798 + 0.069	+ 0.1
ADP	0.578 + 0.056	0.544 + 0.045	- 5.9
AMP	0.051 + 0.003	0.053 + 0.004	+ 3.9
ATP) ADP) AMP)	3.423 + 0.132	3.395 + 0.065	- 0.8
$\frac{ATP}{ADP}$	4.884 + 0.572	5.179 + 0.506	+ 6.0
AEC	0.901 + 0.026	0.904 + 0.007	+ 0.3
Lactate	1.913 + 0.092	1.994 + 0.071*	+ 4.2
Pyruvate	0.117 + 0.009	0.115 + 0.009	- 1.7
$\frac{Lactate}{Pyruvate}$	16.467 + 1.635	17.446 + 1.818	+ 5.9

The values are means of 12 experiments + S.D.
* P < 0.05
AEC = adenylate energy charge

For experimental details see "Materials and Methods".

The results show virtually no change in the cerebral metabolites content, with the
exeption of the slight increase in the lactate concentration, in the brain of hypoxic rats.

Dramatic changes in the cerebral energy metabolism, were observed however in rats
breathing pure nitrogen for only 30 s. The results of these experiments are shown
in Tables 2 and 3. The obtained results are typical for the brain anoxia and show
a dramatic disturbance of the energy metabolism.

ATP, total adenosine nucleotide content, $\frac{ATP}{ADP}$ ratio, adenylate energy charge (AEC),
and creatine phosphate were all decreased significantly. Significant increases of
ADP, AMP and creatine were also observed. The decrease in the concentration of
glycogen, glucose and glucose-6-phosphate was also dramatic.

A significant increase in lactate, pyruvate and lactate/pyruvate ratio was also
observed. NAD[(+)] and NADH were both decreased as was α-ketoglutarate.

No statistically significant changes were observed in the concentrations of citrate, malate, aspartate, glutamate and ammonia.

It appears, therefore, from all data shown on these tables, that 30 s of nitrogen
breathing introduces dramatic changes in the cerebral energy metabolism of the
rat. It should be also mentioned that during 30 s of nitrogen breathing some
change in blood pressure and heart rate was observed. Usually, some decrease in
blood pressure in the first 25 s of nitrogen breathing was observed followed by an
increase at 30 s continued at 40 s. A similar situation was observed for the heart
rate (Fig. 3).

TABLE 2   Influence of 30 s of Nitrogen Breathing on Cerebral
           Energy Reserves and associated Compounds in Rats

Metabolite µmol/g wet tissue	Normoxia	Anoxia	Change in %
ATP	2.835 + 0.091	2.349 + 0.112	- 17.1*
ADP	0.572 + 0.054	0.644 + 0.105	+ 12.6*
AMP	0.052 + 0.006	0.064 + 0.011	+ 23.1*
ATP) ADP) AMP)	3.472 + 0.076	3.057 + 0.066	- 11.9*
$\frac{ATP}{ADP}$	5.012 + 0.505	3.758 + 0.739	- 25.0*
AEC	0.903 + 0.008	0.874 + 0.018	- 3.2*
Creatine Phosphate	4.216 + 0.925	2.519 + 0.532	- 40.2*
Creatine	5.545 + 0.432	6.342 + 0.826	+ 14.4*
Glucose	1.490 + 0.136	0.860 + 0.262	- 42.3*
Glucose-6- Phosphate	0.202 + 0.051	0.119 + 0.047	- 41.1*
Glycogen	3.291 + 0.496	1.942 + 0.442	- 41.0*
Pyruvate	0.100 + 0.011	0.116 + 0.018	+ 16.0*
Lactate	1.816 + 0.235	2.714 + 0.428	+ 49.5*
$\frac{Lactate}{Pyruvate}$	18.299 + 2.755	23.711 + 3.825	+ 29.6*

Values are means of 20 experiments + S.D.

* $P < 0.05$

For experimental details see "Materials and Methods".

V. Stefanovich

TABLE 3   Influence of 30 s of Nitrogen Breathing on some
Cerebral Metabolites of the Rat

Metabolite μmol/g wet tissue	Normoxia	Anoxia	Change in %
NAD$^{(+)}$	0.350 + 0.055	0.312 + 0.079	- 10.8 *
NADH	0.226 + 0.075	0.172 + 0.036	- 23.9 *
$\dfrac{NAD^{(+)}}{NADH}$	1.773 + 0.785	1.934 + 0.718	+ 9.1 NS
NAD$^{(+)}$) / NADH)	0.576 + 0.056	0.484 + 0.069	- 16.0 *
α-Ketoglutarate	0.175 + 0.049	0.099 + 0.035	- 43.4 *
Citrate	0.294 + 0.042	0.282 + 0.045	- 4.1 NS
Malate	0.296 + 0.022	0.312 + 0.060	+ 5.4 NS
Asparate	2.950 + 0.466	3.124 + 0.518	+ 5.9 NS
Glutamate	11.882 + 1.484	12.006 + 1.275	+ 1.0 NS
NH$_4$$^{(+)}$	0.459 + 0.078	0.471 + 0.074	+ 2.6 NS

Values are means of 20 experiments + S.D.
* P < 0.05
For experimental details see "Materials and Methods".

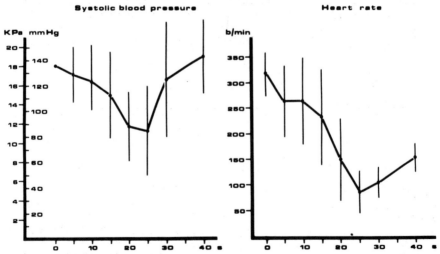

Fig. 3. Influence of 30 s of nitrogen breathing on a systolic
blood pressure and a heart rate of the rat. All points
are averages of seven experiments + S.D.

Change in body temperature as measured by vaginal temperature during 30 s of nitrogen breathing was expressed in a hypothermia reaching the maximum about 9 min
after the beginning of anoxia and amounting to 0.5 °C (Fig. 4).

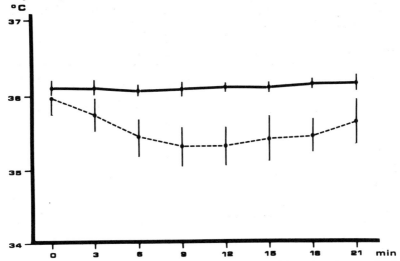

Fig. 4. Influence of 30 s of nitrogen breathing on the vaginal
temperature of a rat; — normal rat, - - experimental
rat. All points are averages of 5 experiments $\pm$ S.E.
Room temperature was 20.5 °C.

The influence of 30 s of nitrogen breathing on blood gases is shown in Table 4.

TABLE 4   Influence of 30 s Nitrogen breathing on Blood Gases
           in the Rat

	Normoxia	Anoxia	P Value
pH	7.420 $\pm$ 0.03	7.510 $\pm$ 0.03	< 0.005
$P_a CO_2$ (mm Hg)	34.1 $\pm$ 4.1	24.7 $\pm$ 2.8	< 0.005
$P_a O_2$ (mm Hg)	96.9 $\pm$ 9.1	20.4 $\pm$ 6.5	< 0.005

Values are means of 10 experiments $\pm$ S.D.
For experimental details see "Materials and Methods".

All changes in pH, P_aCO_2 and P_aO_2 are statistically significant. Especially dramatic was the decrease of P_aO_2 after 30 s of nitrogen breathing. Although the cerebral metabolic change observed in rats after 30 s of nitrogen breathing is substantial, it is apparently not irreversible. The recovery of the cerebral energy metabolism of the rat after breathing nitrogen for 30 s appears to be virtually complete already after five minutes of air breathing subsequent to anoxia. The results
of these experiments are shown in Table 5.

TABLE 5   Influence of 5 min of a Recovery Period after 30 s of
           Nitrogen Breathing on some Cerebral Metabolites in
           the Rat

Metabolite µmol/g wet weight	Normoxia	Anoxia	5 min recovery
ATP	2.859 + 0.098*	2.368 + 0.09	2.851 + 0.12
ADP	0.591 + 0.046	0.682 + 0.05	0.533 + 0.02
AMP	0.053 + 0.005	0.067 + 0.005	0.054 + 0.005
ATP) ADP) AMP)	3.526 + 0.080	3.116 + 0.12	3.438 + 0.13
$\frac{ATP}{ADP}$	4.899 + 0.413	3.489 + 0.24	5.357 + 0.36
AEC	0.901 + 0.006	0.869 + 0.006	0.907 + 0.004
Lactate	1.910 + 0.158	2.592 + 0.06	2.795 + 0.14**
Pyruvate	0.103 + 0.010	0.119 + 0.006	0.095 + 0.010
$\frac{Lactate}{Pyruvate}$	18.595 + 2.176	21.890 + 1.1	29.799 + 7.1 **

* Mean of 10 experiments + S.D.

** P < 0.005 when normoxia group and 5 min recovery group were
   compared.

For experimental details see "Materials and Methods".

The results show that already after five minutes of the recovery period, virtually
no significant change in the cerebral metabolites of the experimental group are
present, when compared with the control group. The only significant change left,
is the increased concentration of lactate and the lactate/pyruvate ratio.
Thirty seconds of nitrogen breathing has also a profound effect on the cyclic nucleotide systems. The results of such experiments are shown in Table 6. The results
presented in this table show that after 30 s of nitrogen breathing there is a
significant increase in cAMP as the result of a simultaneous activation of adena-
late cyclase and a decrease in cAMP PDE activity. This decrease in cAMP PDE activity is obvious only if investigated immediately after anoxia.
It can be mentioned that these results offer an explanation for the decrease in
glycogen observed in our experiments. Increased concentration of cAMP resulting
from anoxia activates the enzyme protein kinase which activates phosphorylase b
kinase. As a consequence, phosphorylase b is converted into phosphorylase a, with
a resulting breakdown of glycogen.

The change in the cGMP concentration is in the opposite direction to the change in the
cAMP concentration. This decrease in the cGMP content is the result of the decrease in the guanylate cyclase activity. Change in cGMP PDE activity was not significant. In 1975 Goldberg and others have suggested that the cellular control
mechanisms in bidirectionally regulated systems are mediated through the opposing
action of cGMP and cAMP.
This dualism hypothesis does not seem to be valid in all situations, however in
our experiments with anoxic rats, the Yin - Yang hypothesis seems to be valid.

TABLE 6   The Influence of 30 s of Nitrogen Breathing on Cyclic
           Nucleotides Systems in Rat Brain

Metabolite or activity	n	normal rats	anoxic rats	change in %	statistical significance
cAMP pmol/mg tissue	40	1.15 + 0.38*	1.76 + 0.67	+ 53	P < 0.005
Adenylate cyclase pmol/mg protein/min	21	48.60 + 9.10	55.70 + 8.40	+ 14.6	P < 0.02
cGMP pmol/mg tissue	11	0.051 + 0.008	0.043 + 0.007	- 15.7	P < 0.005
Guanylate cyclase pmol/mg protein/min	11	23.33 + 1.60	21.03 + 1.30	- 9.8	P < 0.01
cAMP PDE activity nmol/mg protein/min (s) = 1.0 mM	8	21.5 + 4.7	17.8 + 2.4	- 17.2	P < 0.025
cGMP PDE activity nmol/mg protein/min (s) = 0.1 μM	8	1.53 + 0.13	1.49 + 0.10	- 2.6	NS

* mean + S.D.

For experimental details see "Materials and Methods".

DISCUSSION

The rat brain can withstand a moderate degree of hypoxia for a relatively long
time. In our experiments at 10 % oxygen for a week, normal concentrations of cerebral ATP, ADP, and AMP were present and a steady state corresponding to a normal
adenylate energy charge (0.904) was maintained (Table 1). The sudden exposure of
the rat to 100 % nitrogen atmosphere for 30 s caused a significant change of cerebral energy metabolism as shown by Ridge (1972). In our experiments rat brain
could no longer maintain a high AEC of 0.903 (Table 2), which after 30 s of nitrogen breathing decreased for 3.2 % to 0.874. It should be mentioned, however, that
our results show the level of AEC in the whole brain. It is possible that more metabolically active areas of the brain attain during anoxia lower AEC values and
less metabolically ative areas exhibit somewhat higher AEC values. This could explain why some regions of a brain are selectively vulnerable to the lack of
oxygen.
A significant decrease in the content of total adenine nucleotides was also observed in rats brain after breathing nitrogen for 30 s (Table 2). This could be eventually explained rather by a decreased rate of synthesis than by an increased rate
of degradation, as cerebral ATP, which activate AMP deaminase (Weil-Malherbe and
Green, 1955) is also very much diminished.

Comparing all cerebral metabolites, the highest decrease, in percents of normal value, was observed for α-ketoglutarate. The similar situation was noted by Norberg and Siesjö (1975) in their study of changes in pyruvate and citric acid cycle intermediate in rat cerebral cortex after one min of exposure to a hypoxic gas mixture (P_a O_2 about 25 mm Hg).

Lactate was the metabolite which increased to the highest level (+ 49.5 %) as a result of 30 s anoxia (Table 2). Pyruvate increased also, but to a lower extent (+ 16.0 %). Accordingly the lactate/pyruvate ratio has significantly increased (+ 29.6 %). The decreases in the concentrations of NADH (-23.0 %) and $NAD^{(+)}$ (- 10.8 %) were also significant. Calculation of the free cytoplasmic $NAD^{(+)}$/NADH ratio after the method of Krebs and Veech (1970) shows the decrease of this parameter from 495 (normoxia) to 384 (anoxia).

This decrease in the cytoplasmic $NAD^{(+)}$/NADH ratio is not favorable, because a high ratio is necessary to allow a high forward flux through the glyceraldehyde phosphate dehydrogenase step in a complete oxydation of glucose.

Concerning the influence of 30 s of nitrogen breathing on cyclic nucleotide systems in rat brain, our results show an increase in the cAMP level and a decrease in the cGMP concentration. These data, explained as a result of corresponding enzymatic activities are supporting Yin Yang hypothesis of Goldberg and others (1975). It can be suggested that the increased concentration of AMP as a result of 30 s of nitrogen breathing is leading to an increased level of adenosine formed from AMP by the enzyme 5'-nucleotidase. Adenosine, bound to the receptor is stimulating adenylate cyclase, causing an increase of cAMP. In order to explain the effect of anoxia on cyclic nucleotide systems of rat brain, a recent study concerning the influence of theophylline on cAMP and cGMP level in rat brain should be mentioned (Stefanovich, 1979).

Theophylline is a reasonable good inhibitor of rat brain cAMP and cGMP PDE's and a somewhat besser inhibitor of cAMP PDE than of cGMP PDE.

In vivo situation mirror these in vitro findings, but only when the concentration of theophylline is high enough (e.g. 100 mg/kg p.o.). Then, some increase in cAMP and cGMP content can be observed. Only the increase in cAMP was statistically significant. It is also generally assumed as the result of several studies (Satin and Rall 1970, Mah and Daly 1976 and Green and Stanberry 1977) that theophylline competes with adenosine released as a result of e.g. hypoxia. Adenosine is an activator of adenylate cyclase and theophylline is not - as the result, a relative decrease in cAMP level is observed after e.g. incubation of brain slices with theophylline (Mah and Daly 1976). In results of in vivo experiments shown in the Fig. 5 it can be seen that, as previously observed, anoxia increases the rat brain cAMP content and decreases the cGMP level. It can be also noted that in normal rats, theophylline increases cAMP and cGMP levels in the rat brain. The increase of the former cyclic nucleotide is more significant than the increase of the latter.

The influence of theophylline in anoxic rat brain is expressed in a significant decrease in the cAMP level and in a significant increase in cGMP level.

The opposing effect of theophylline on cAMP and cGMP concentrations in the anoxic rat brain is difficult to explain. A hypothetical explanation for this phenomenon is offered in Fig. 6.

In the cell membrane an adenosine receptor is connected with adenylate cyclase, which is further linked with a guanylate cyclase. The increased concentration of adenosine e.g. produced as the result of anoxia, is changing the conformation of adenylate cyclase in such a way that adenylate cyclase is activated. The changed conformation of adenylate cyclase is producing a change in the conformation of guanylate cyclase. This change, however, is expressed in a decrease of activity of the latter enzyme.

When the anoxic rat has obtained a relatively large amount of theophylline (e.g. 100 mg/kg p.o.), the effect of anoxia is diminished as a result of competition between adenosine and theophylline. This is reflected in a decrease of adenylate cyclase activity leading to normalized cyclic nucleotide levels in the rat brain. We

have observed this phenomenon not only with theophylline, but also with several
other xanthines. The same xanthines were also active in decreasing the effect of
anoxia on adenine nucleotides.

All here presented experimental data show that exposing rat to nitrogen breathing
for 30 s produces dramatic changes in the energy metabolism and the metabolism of
cyclic nucleotide in rat brain. Data are reproducible and easy to obtain.

It can be suggested therefore, that the anoxic rat model could be used in a
search for a potential antihypoxic drug.

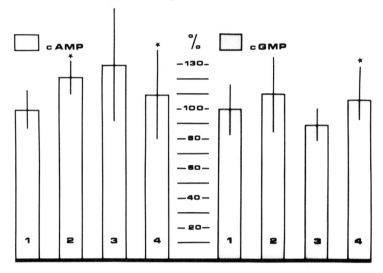

Fig. 5. cAMP and cGMP content in brain of normal and anoxic
        rats one hour after administration of theophylline
        (100 mg/kg p.o.).

        1 = normoxia, 2 = normoxia + theophylline,
        3 = anoxia, 4 = anoxia + theophylline.

        * = statistically significant at $P < 0.05$.
            Theophylline samples were always compared with
            control samples.

        n = 10   Adapted from Stefanovich, 1979.

122   V. Stefanovich

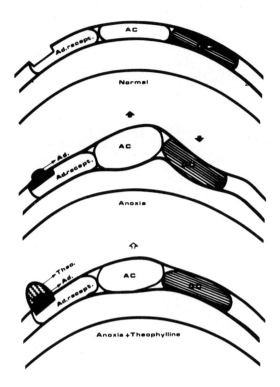

Fig. 6. Schematic presentation of the influence of
        theophylline on the adenosine receptor -
        adenylate cyclase - guanylate cyclase system in
        rat brain membranes.

        Ad = adenosine, AC = adenylate cyclase, GC =
        guanylate cyclase, Theo = theophylline.

REFERENCES

Atkinson, D. E. (1968).The energy charge of the adenylate pool as regulatory
    parameter. Interaction with feed-back modifiers. Biochemistry, 7, 4030-4034.
Bergmeyer, H. U. (1974). Methoden der enzymatischen Analyse. Verlag Chemie,
    Weinheim.
Goldberg, N. D., M. K. Haddox, S. E. Nicol, D. B. Glass, C. H. Sanford, F. A. Kuehl,
    Jr., and R. Estensen (1975). Biological regulation through opposing influences
    of cyclic GMP and cyclic AMP: the Yin Yang hypothesis, in G. I. Drummond,
    P. Greengard and G. A. Robison (eds.), Advances in Cyclic Nucleotide Research,
    Vol. 5, Raven Press, New York.
Gornall, A. C., J. C. Bardowill, and M. M. David (1949). Determination of serum
    proteins by means of the biuret reaction. J. biol. Chem., 177, 751-766.
Green, R. D., and L. R.Stanberry (1977). Elevation of cyclic AMP in C-1300 murine
    neuroblastoma by adenosine and related compounds and the antagonism of this res-
    ponse by methylxanthines. Biochem. Pharmacol., 26, 37-43.
Krebs, H. A., and R. L. Veech (1970). Regulation of the redox state of the pyridine
    nucleotides in rat liver, in H. Sund (Ed.), Pyridine Nucleotide-dependent Dehy-
    drogenases, Springer Verlag, Berlin, pp. 413-434.

McMillan, V., and B. K. Siesjö (1972). Brain energy metabolism in hypoxia, Scand. J. clin. Lab. Invest., 30, 127-136.

Mah, H. D., and J. W. Daly (1976). Adenosine-dependent formation of cyclic AMP in brain slices. Pharmacol. Res. Commun., 8, 65-79.

Norberg, K., and B. K. Siesjö (1975). Cerebral metabolism in hypoxic hypoxia. II. Cyclic acid cycle intermediates and associated amino acids. Brain Res., 86, 45-54.

Pichard, A. L., and W. Y. Cheung (1976). Cyclic 3',5'nucleotide phosphodiesterase. Interconvertible multiple forms and their effects on enzyme activity and kinetics. J. Biol. Chem., 251, 5726-5737.

Ridge, J. W. (1972). Hypoxia and the energy charge of the cerebral adenylate pool. Biochem. J., 127, 351-355.

Satin, A., and T. W. Rall (1970). The effect of adenosine and adenine nucleotides on the cyclic adenosine 3',5'-phosphate content of guinea pig cerebral cortex slices. Mol. Pharmacol., 6, 13-23.

Shier, W., H. Baldwin, M. Nilsen-Hamilton, T. Hamilton, and M. Thanassi (1976). Regulation of guanylate and adenylate cyclase activities by lysolecithin. Proc. Natl. Acad. Sci. USA, 73, 1586-1590.

Siesjö, B. K. (1977). Physiological aspects of brain energy metabolism, in A. N. Davison (Ed.), Biochemical Correlates of Brain Structure and Function, Academic Press, New York, p.p. 175-213.

Stefanovich, V. (1979). Influence of theophylline on concentrations of cyclic 3',5'-adenosine monophosphate and cyclic 3'5'-guanosine monophosphate of rat brain. Neurochem. Res., 4, 587-594.

Veech, R. L., R. L. Harris, D. Veloso, and E. H. Veech (1973). Freeze-blowing: a new technique for the study of brain in vivo. J. Neurochem., 20, 183-188.

Weil-Malherbe, H., and R. H. Green (1955). Ammonia formation in brain. I. Studies on slices and suspensions. Biochem. J., 61, 210-218.

124   V. Stefanovich

DISCUSSION

Schraven: After which time lactate returned to normal?

Stefanovich: We did check the concentration of metabolites only after five
minutes of recovery. At the time lactate was still significantly increased.

Sokoloff: I would imagine that 30 seconds of breathing with nitrogen will turn
on the number of pathways in the brain and alter activities in specific regions
that could affect adenylate cyclase activity?

Stefanovich: Yes, adenylate cyclase activity was significantly increased, most
likely due to increased adenosine.

Hossmann: Is there also a normalization of cAMP or adenylate cyclase after
5 minutes of recovery?

Stefanovich: After 5 minutes of recovery we did study only adenine nucleotide
content.

Sokoloff: Any other subjects to be brought for discussion? Then, I guess, we come
to the end of the programme. I found it a very stimulating programme. I learnt a
good deal and we had more questions than answers. But that's the way we have to
go for the future. What we need in this field, I think, are new ideas, new
questions that we can examine by new methods and I think it's still a long way off
before we find a way to help the damaged brain.

I would like to thank Prof. Stefanovich and Prof. Krieglstein and the people from
Hoechst Laboratories for inviting us, for having organized this meeting, and I
would like to express my thanks to all colleagues participating in the discussion.
I am sure that everybody else here would like to do the same.

Stefanovich: In the name of Prof. Krieglstein and Dr. Wolf, and in my own name I
would like to thank our chairmen Prof. Mandel and Prof. Sokoloff and all participants for the success of this meeting.

INDEX

The page numbers refer to the first page of the contribution in which the index term appears.

ATP   75
Adenine nucleotides   75
Adenylate energy change (EC)   19
Amphetamines   1
Anoxia   87
  rat model   111
Artificial blood   19
Auditory deprivation   1
Auditory system   1
Autoradiographic technique   1

Blood flow   47
  cortical   65
Brain   75
  edema   47
  fuels of   87
  human   87
  insect   87
  metabolism   1
    anaerobic   87
    energy   19, 35, 47, 87, 111
  perfusion   19
  swelling   47
γ-Butyrolactone   1

Carbon dioxide   1, 87
Carotid artery, ligation   47
Cats   47
Cephalopods   87
Cerebral artery occlusion   47
Cerebral functional activity   1
Cerebro-vascular disease   47
Cholinergic innervation   65
Cortex   1
  visual   1
Cyanide   35

Dementia   35

Deoxyglucose   1
$[^{14}C]$ Deoxyglucose method   1
Deoxyglucose-6-phosphatase   1
2-Deoxyglucose-6-phosphate (DG-6-P)   1
2,4-Dinitrophenol   35
Diving   87

EEG   19
Edema   47
Electron microscopy   75
Endoplasmatic reticulum, rough   35
Energy metabolism, brain   19, 35, 47, 87, 111
Enzyme activity   75
Eye ball   47

Fatty acids, oxidation   87
Fructose-1, 6-diphosphate   19, 35

Gerontopsychiatric disorders   35
^{3}H-Glucose   87
Glucose-6-phosphatase   1
Glucose utilization   1
Glycogen   87
Glycolysis   19

Hexokinase   1, 87
High-energy phosphates   19
Honey bees   87
Hydrogen clearance method   65
γ-Hydroxybutyrate   1
Hypercapnia   65
Hypocapnia   65
Hypoxia   87
  chronic   75
  energy metabolism of brain   87
  10% O_2 111
  rat model   111

126   Index

Inferior colliculus 1
Ischemia 19, 47
  thresholds of 47
Ischemic blood edema 7
Isonicotinic acid hydrozide (INH) 35

Ketone bodies 87

Lactate dehydrogenase 75
  activity 75
  bound 75
  iso-enzymes 75
  soluble 75
  of synaptosomes 75
Lumped constant 1
d-Lysergic acid diethylamide 1

Maxwell equation 47
Metabolic rates 87
Myelin 75
Metamphetamine 35
Methohexital 19
Microsphere 47
Middle cerebral artery occlusion 47
Morphine 1

Naloxone 1
Nerve fibres
  adrenergic 65
  cholinergic 65
Nitrogen breathing 111

Octopine 87
Ocular dominance columns 1
Oxygen consumption 87

Penicillin 1
Perfusion medium, fluorocarbon 19
Phlorizin 35
Phosphofructokinase 19, 35, 87
Pial arteries 65
Polysomes 35

Rats 75
Rhesus monkey 1

Sciatic nerve 1
Seizures 1
Sodium/potassium ratio 47
Spontaneously hypertensive rats 47
Starvation 87
Stroke, experimental 47
Subcellular distribution 75
Superior cervical ganglion 65
Sympathectomy 65

Therapy 47
Thiopental 1
Triton X-100 75

Vertebrates and invertebrates 87
Vincristine 35